What Is Medicine?

The publisher gratefully acknowledges the generous support of the Sue Tsao Endowment Fund in Chinese Studies of the University of California Press Foundation.

What Is Medicine?

WESTERN AND EASTERN
APPROACHES TO HEALING

PAUL U. UNSCHULD

Translated from the German by Karen Reimers

UNIVERSITY OF CALIFORNIA PRESS
Berkeley   Los Angeles   London

University of California Press, one of the most distinguished
university presses in the United States, enriches lives around
the world by advancing scholarship in the humanities, social
sciences, and natural sciences. Its activities are supported by
the UC Press Foundation and by philanthropic contributions
from individuals and institutions. For more information, visit
www.ucpress.edu.

University of California Press
Berkeley and Los Angeles, California

University of California Press, Ltd.
London, England

Library of Congress Cataloging-in-Publication Data

Unschuld, Paul U. (Paul Ulrich).
   [Was ist Medizin? English]
   What is medicine? : Western and Eastern approaches to healing /
Paul U. Unschuld ; translated from the German by Karen Reimers.
       p.   cm.
   Includes index.
   ISBN 978-0-520-25765-8 (cloth : alk. paper)
   ISBN 978-0-520-25766-5 (pbk. : alk. paper)
      1. Medicine—Philosophy—History.   2. Medicine, Oriental—
Philosophy—History.   I. Title.
      [DNLM: 1. Philosophy, Medical.   2. Cross-Cultural Comparison.
3. Medicine, East Asian Traditional.   w 61 U59 2009]

R723.U56   2009
610.1—dc22

Manufactured in the United States of America

18   17   16   15   14   13   12   11   10   09
10   9   8   7   6   5   4   3   2   1

This book is printed on Cascades Enviro 100, a 100% post consumer
waste, recycled, de-inked fiber. FSC recycled certified and processed
chlorine free. It is acid free, Ecologo certified, and manufactured by
BioGas energy.

To Charles Leslie,
friend and mentor.

Plausibility is the brother of truth.

Contents

Preface

Everyone experiences illness at some point. If we can no longer help ourselves as laypeople, we turn to medicine. In such cases, we trust in the medical interpretation of our illness. This interpretation is normally a complex theoretical edifice. It serves to explain the healthy and diseased states of the human organism. But how do such theoretical edifices come into being? Can a shrewd observer identify the core functions of the body merely by looking at it? Does the body have sufficient force of expression to disclose to us the explanations backing up medical thought and practice?

The answer to these questions is offered by the past two millennia of Western and Chinese medicine: fundamental theories about the functioning of the human organism cannot have arisen solely from observation of the body. The image we construct of the body invariably requires a model external to that body. Stimuli for interpretations of the human organism always originate in life experience and in an actual or desired living environment. A medical theory is plausible if it mirrors our own life experience and an actual or desired living environment, simultaneously integrating knowledge of the body's verifiable structures.

This book depicts the fascinating development of medical thought in West and East. It shows for the first time, continuously for both civilizations, the close bond between medical thought and the prevailing social and economic conditions governing man's living environment. Surprisingly, there is a far-reaching, cross-cultural parallelism of traditions spanning two millennia. Why did "Western medicine," grounded in European culture, find such an enthusiastic reception in China in the nineteenth and twentieth centuries? Will "Chinese medicine" gain long-term importance as a dynamic, independent form of alternative therapy in China and in the Western world? Can the development of medical thought be directed or regulated? Can health policy dictate a single system of medical ideas for everyone? What are the effects of globalization on medical thought? The statements in this book offer suggestions to help answer these questions.

1 | Life = Body Plus X

Let us assume the following. We want to understand the functions of the human body. Then, we want to explain these functions to other people. Where do we begin? What does the body disclose to us? A fair amount. Our senses tell us much: there is color in the face and on the body, seen with our eyes. There are odors that we smell with our nose. There are sounds in the chest and the abdomen that we hear with our ears. None of this is static; it is always changing, day and night, in times of health and illness. We see that food is absorbed in the body and then excreted in an altered form. The body surface is sometimes dry. Following exertion, in frightened states, and during fever, sweat comes out of the pores. Fever shows that temperature also fluctuates. Skin can break open, and a wound can also close up again. Hair grows and falls out. Tears flow and dry up. The body discloses a fair amount to us.

We do not have to restrict our observation to the living body. The dead also disclose a fair amount to us. In an opened corpse, in addition to the external organs that we can see in a living person—the nose, eyes, ears, and mouth—there are also the internal organs. Here again we see colors, outlines, fluids. A fair amount is offered to the senses. But is that all? And what is it all there for? How does the whole thing work? There are conditions that prevent us from pursuing our daily activities. We denote some of these conditions as "illness." We would like to know why such conditions arise. For that, we must know what is "healthy." There are various criteria for separating the "normal" from the "abnormal" and the healthy from the sick.

Then there is another problem. Humans, like every living organism, have a material body. But at the same time, there is also something intangible, which is life itself. The body seems to be directed by life. Life can escape a person, and his or her body ceases to function. Thus, in our endeavor to understand ourselves and our functions, we already have three levels. We perceive the material body. We assume that in this material body, certain processes occur that we can classify as normal or abnormal. Then there is also a directing level. Something directs the body in its functions. Something is responsible for certain processes occurring in the body. The body can lose this "something." Then it dies. But what is this "something"?

We cannot see it. But it has many names—a different one in every culture. The designations have also changed through the ages. Let us focus on the human body and simply take from the multitude of designations a commonly used name for the invisible something: the spirit. We could also say soul. We assume that the body cannot live without a soul. The soulless body exists only as a dead body. It makes no difference whether we speak of body and spirit, body and soul or *corpus* and *spiritus*. One thing we can see, the other we cannot.

The assumption of the existence of a spirit, a soul, a *spiritus* in the body is a first indication: when we speak of the human body and its functions, we must fall back on ideas that do not originate in what we can see in a tangible substrate, or in the conceivability of matter, whatever its nature. An endeavor to explain certain functions of the body, and with that to explain certain human behaviors, inevitably leads to the assumption of invisible, intangible, but nevertheless real parts of the living body. What is the basis for this assumption? Possibly a comparison of the living body with the dead body.

Viewing a peacefully dying or newly deceased person, one can hardly see any difference between life and death. Death first appears as sleep; only the act of touching the dead person and the further development of the corpse show us that death is another state. Yet there is no doubt: the corpse seems to be missing something; something seems to have escaped from the dead body. What is now missing once gave the person the ability to live. It is not visible or tangible.

The observed death is not necessarily accompanied by a loss of blood. It is even the rule that no material, tangible substrate leaves the living body at death. Today, we still do not know exactly what threshold separates life from death, what element of life must be lost for death to occur. Even in prehistoric times—though the exact origin is unknown—the formula already seemed plausible: life is a body augmented by X.

So far, the identification of X has come no further than an assumption, a construction. When we speak of the "soul," the "spirit," or the "psyche," we use metaphors. For example, the soul can be "dirtied" or "black," and should be "pure." Such a statement, for many centuries associated with very real circumstances, likely seems to many today to have validity only as a metaphor. However, today's same enlightened thinkers will unabashedly acknowledge contemporary derivations of X, in accordance with which the "psyche" is "vulnerable" and should be "protected from harm." It is no use: the soul, psyche, spirit, or whatever else we have called X or want to call it seems to be a necessary element of life, an indispensable attendant to the living body. If we want to explain the functions of the living body, we cannot do without X, the invisible, the intangible. At least not yet.

The names for X are adapted to their context of interpretation, sometimes religious, sometimes secular. Certain conventions can impress themselves in a cultural context. Referring merely to "X" is not sophisticated enough. Better to speak of $X_1, X_2 \ldots X_n$. Let us call X_1 "soul," which is responsible for different functions than X_2, which we call "spirit." X_3, "psyche," is in turn responsible for different functions than X_1 and X_2. Further differentiations are not out of the question. The ethereal and astral parts of the body, so clear to students of Rudolf Steiner, are differentiations of X. Likewise, the construction of *qi*, now widely accepted in Europe and North America, was conceptualized in its Chinese homeland about two millennia ago as a fine material breath, and has now contributed in the West to a further differentiation of the invisible X into a kind of life force or energy. Today, the life formula therefore needs to be corrected. The precise formula is now: life is a body augmented by $X_1, X_2, X_3 \ldots X_n$. Whether every X, as the many names seem to suggest, actually exists alongside the others, or whether X_1 to X_n are actually all just one single X for which we know no comprehensive name or do not dare to name, all of this remains unknown. X is X, after all.

Everything points to this: the loss of the ability to participate in daily life unhindered; the loss of the ability to accomplish one's tasks and to fulfill routine duties appropriate to one's place in the arc from birth through adulthood to the end of life. This was the earliest criterion for the identification of the condition categorized as "illness." Today, there is a more differentiated perspective. We differentiate between underlying diseases on the one hand, and visible or tangible ailments on the other. An invisible disease can be the cause of a visible or tangible ailment. Fever is consequently not a disease in itself; it is an expression, a symptom of a more profound disease. The underlying disease is not necessarily detectable by the patient—at least not in the beginning stages. Thus the disease hypertension, for example.

Even in very early times, there was a differentiation between illness of the tangible, visible body and illness of X, the intangible, invisible spirit. X, as we have seen, is hidden from perception by the eye and other sensory organs, but it actually exists. It is so real to us that we grant that X can be healthy or sick—just as the body can.

If the body is in a condition that prevents us from fulfilling our daily tasks, for instance when we have a high fever or a broken leg, then it is sick. If the body is apparently unharmed, but a person's behavior is such that he is unable to fulfill his daily tasks, then X is sick. To illustrate this, let us again give X a name. We refer to people as being "insane," "mentally ill," and "emotionally disturbed." What is actually supposed to be ill when we say "the psyche is ill"? No one knows. It is an assumption, a construct stemming from the parallel to harm of the body, which can be ill. It is possible that something else is behind "diseases of the spirit," something much different from what we can presently imagine. There is no discernible short- or long-term way out of the dichotomy between the comprehensible and the incomprehensible, between the physically tangible and the intellectual construct.

Let there be no doubt: both the body and X can be healthy or sick. At the same time, a healthy body can accommodate a sick X and vice versa. Since antiquity, observers of human life have been convinced that a sick body can cause an initially healthy X to fall ill, just as an initially sick X can subsequently cause the body to fall ill. Depending on the direction of this process, we speak of psychosomatics or somatopsychics. These terms summarize what this is all about. Reality *(soma)* and speculation *(psyche)* are linked in one word, as if this were a matter of two partners of the same rank. And they are in fact partners—only death can separate the body and X. It is a widely held misconception that Descartes was the first to separate body and soul. It is true that his physiological ideas shone new light on the separation of body and soul in a different way than any thinker before him. But the first separation took place millennia beforehand, at a time when the body and X were given different names. And that is an event that can be traced back to antiquity.

Very early on, the idea emerged that a body and its X could seem totally normal or healthy to the naïve observer, but still be classified by experts as sick or abnormal. Perhaps the oldest record of this conceptual expansion is found in the *Records of the Grand Historian* of Sima Qian, written at the turn of the second to first century BC in China. In his history of ancient China, Sima Qian included a biography of the itinerant physician Bian Que. When he was first admitted for an audience with Marquis Huan of Qi, Bian Que at once informed the marquis that the latter was sick and required treatment. Neither the marquis nor his royal household suspected any illness., and the marquis replied tersely that he was not sick. The rest of the story has been recounted many times. It ends with the death of the marquis and the itinerant physician's explanation of the hidden course of illness.

In ancient times, being able to detect a disease invisible to laymen that did not hinder the sick person from pursuing his daily business but was nevertheless present was clearly an exceptional skill. Today it is hardly worth mentioning, since it happens every day. The body can be sick with hypertension, without the patient or his neighbor noticing any reduction in his fitness or any behavioral change. The body can be sick with a hidden tumor growing deep in a lung, without the affected person having any discomfort.

Bian Que detected the marquis' illness, and today's physician can diagnose hypertension or early lung cancer, because of something at their disposal that was unavailable to their predecessors: a theory of the processes in the body. This theory is medicine. Only the emergence of medicine could make it possible to recognize early processes in the body as "pathological." At an early stage, it is not any interference with the body's daily efficiency that leads these processes to be called pathological; thus, these processes do not fulfill the first criterion of illness. They are classified as pathological because the expert knows something the layman doesn't.

The physician, with his or her theoretical education, is able to predict the way that these processes, invisible to the untrained eye, will eventually develop so that the original criterion of illness will be fulfilled and the body (and perhaps also X) will be partially or completely deprived of the ability to function.

2 | Medicine, or Novelty Appeal

We can now ask the central question that will concern us for the rest of this book: What is medicine? What provides the theoretical foundations for Bian Que in ancient China to make his prediction, or for today's physician to make his or her evaluations?

Medicine is nothing but the endeavor to understand the normal and abnormal states of the body and of X in their origins and development, to attain the knowledge that is required to promote the normal or healthy states, to prevent the abnormal or sick states, and if a sick state has arisen, to alleviate its effects or even to reverse them completely. All this serves to preserve life, so that a person feels well and can accomplish his daily tasks to the fullest possible extent.

To attain this knowledge, medicine uses the scientific study of nature— the nature of man and his habitat. The science of nature, in turn, is based on the assumption of laws of nature that are valid independently of time, space, and person. As such, medicine is merely a part of healing. Healing is the overarching concept. Healing includes all efforts to heal the body and X or to preserve health. These might be prayers to a god or gods, exorcism of demons, massage, or administration of substances known to influence certain functions of the body. Healing of this kind is not medicine. Healing becomes medicine only when its practitioners recognize laws of nature and use only these laws of nature to investigate possible explanations of the body's functions.

Healing is, generally speaking, the endeavor to prevent abnormal states of the body and to treat them if they occur. Healing can consist merely in performing a healing activity, such as cooling a hot place on the body. No theory is needed for this. It is pure empiricism. However, healing can also have a theoretical, interpretive aspect. If a certain type of healing is to be considered medicine, then the interpretive part of this healing relies solely on the laws of nature for its interpretations. With nonmedical healing, the interpretive part may be based on the numinous, that is, on the existence of spirits, gods, ancestors, or a single god.

Medicine is a relatively young cultural construct. Healing has existed since the prehistoric era; its beginnings are lost in the darkness of a time from when no documents remain. In ancient Egypt, healing existed, but not medicine. Today, healing is still pursued in manifold ways. Only a part of all healing efforts today can be considered medical. Much is undertaken without the known laws of nature being used as the guiding principle. Medicine in Europe began to emerge around the fifth or fourth century BC. At the other end of the Eurasian continent, in China, medicine also emerged two or three centuries later out of the older healing. It is not yet known whether there was a relationship between these two events.

The emergence of medicine from healing seems to be a logical development. People in antiquity, so we read in the conventional history books, discovered laws of nature and immediately applied these to the functions of the body—and voilà, medicine was born. It sounds convincing, and yet it is not convincing at all. First of all, why should anyone have questioned the previous healing? Did it not offer an explanation for everything? If someone got sick, either the gods or the ancestors had sent the ailment. Perhaps as retribution for human lapses. Countless prayers to the gods or ancestors for forgiveness had brought the desired recovery and reattainment of health. Illnesses that led to death despite prayers were one's unavoidable fate. In those cases, the wrath of the gods or the ancestors was too severe for human sacrifices and pleas to have an easing effect. It is also not as if the other type of healing was relegated hopelessly to the background and forever repressed into oblivion following the emergence of the new medicine. It was quite the opposite, as with the healing cult of Asclepius, which recommended healing sleep on the temple grounds, during which the god himself visited the sick and freed them of their suffering. This cult and many other methods of nonmedical healing came into being only after the emergence of medicine.

One could object that at its beginning, medicine was still helpless in the face of so many problems that it could not prove itself to be a 100-percent-effective alternative to the antiquated forms of healing. This objection, incidentally valid even today—and we will need to return to this—should give us pause. From the healing considered effective for centuries, if not millennia (why else would it have been practiced?), an alternative method developed, one that was *initially* hardly more effective than the already known healing methods.

Given the fact that today every scientifically trained physician would dismiss most of the supposedly effective remedies and methods described in the documents of this "young medicine" as senseless, one wonders what the novelty appeal of the new medicine was. It could not have been its convincing clinical effectiveness. If we look at this carefully, we can determine a first principle of medicine here: novelty appeal in medicine does not follow from proof of clinical effectiveness, but from other stimuli. We need to identify these stimuli if we want to understand the history of medicine—then and now.

Of course, when talking about novelty appeal, we are not referring to new substances or operative techniques discovered through intense research, or chance discoveries aiming to have effects that would make sense to anyone and which are therefore immediately convincing. With novelty appeal, we mean the new thinking, the great new attempt to explain why people are healthy or sick, and following this attempt at explanation, the measures recommended to protect health or to heal sickness. Such great ruptures are more infrequent than one might assume considering that there is more than two thousand years in the history of medicine.

We can also mention a second aspect of novelty appeal. Even within an accepted, dominant model of explanation, fundamentally new thoughts can arise and find acceptance. Examples of such novelties on the second level include the emergence of bacteriology in the late nineteenth century and the emphasis on the role of the immune system in the second half of the twentieth century. We must always ask ourselves where the novelty appeal of the time lay.

But let us stay with antiquity for the time being. The clinical application of the new medicine could not have been so convincing at first—it could not have justified the radical upheaval and the urgency with which its new advocates defended their views. One might have expected humility, modesty. We might expect the authors of the time to have argued something like this: "We believe in the gods, and praying to the gods often helps us heal our patients." Or: "We know about the importance of the ancestors, and the petitions to the ancestors to relieve us of our suffering are often helpful. But now we have the help of an additional new method that we want to use in cases where it has shown itself to be useful and effective and where the former methods fail."

Some people may have thought and acted this way. More than a few people take action this way even today. Yet these people are not those who are responsible for what is new. People who think and act this pragmatically are hangers-on, beneficiaries, not the proponents of what is new, not creators. The creators of what is new speak a different language. They think only in terms of either/or. The creators disdain the old; they are interested only in what is new. Where does this deep conviction come from? Since it is not derived from the clinical effectiveness of the new thinking, it must have another source. Once we find this source, we will know the stimulus for what is fundamentally new in medicine.

Let us explore the two ancient cultures for which there is ancient evidence that can be dated quite precisely, documenting the emergence of medicine from the healing that had long been known.

3 | Why Laws of Nature?

In China, medicine developed in the early second century BC, a time that was well removed from the beginning of the historical era and well documented. Rich source material gives us a good idea of the previous era. We are familiar with healing in China, out of which and against the backdrop of which Chinese medicine developed. In the present state of research, we can also redraw the beginnings of science, the precondition for the emergence of medicine in the narrower sense defined above.

Let us start with the emergence of science in China. The essence of science lies in the assumption that inherent laws determine all events in the universe—irrespective of place, time, and person. He who assumes such inherent laws must initially pay a high price. He must defend himself against those who maintain that events are the more or less arbitrary work of gods, ancestors, or demons.

From time immemorial, knowledge of the power of the gods, ancestors, and demons determined much of human individual and social interaction. The gods were capable of intervening in the course of events, of sending rain or punishing with drought, of making a harvest possible or destroying it, of imposing death on a person or allowing someone to recover from illness. And was there not enough evidence to prove that this knowledge corresponded to reality? Hadn't prayers, if they just lasted long enough, often brought the desired rain? Hadn't sacrifices ended the series of bad harvests? Did not father recover from his grave illness, despite his high fever, once the demons had been expelled with the proper methods? Anecdotal evidence. There weren't any precise statistics then; the appearance of many cases sufficed.

So why risk radical change? This was no mere matter of opinion, it was a matter of power—hard, political power. Those who positioned themselves between the people and the gods, those who claimed to know the will of the gods or ancestors, promulgated detailed rules on how people should live—rules that bestowed benefits on the mediators themselves. The interpretation of misfortune, or the wish to influence a future event in one way or another with the help of the numinous powers, brought advantages to those who declared themselves mediators and knew the right prayers—advantages that amounted to power. Through the mediators' pronouncements on the demands of the gods, spirits, and demons, the supplicants' behavior could be controlled and certain social structures were consolidated.

All this was called into question by the conviction that events in the world are controlled by laws, not by the arbitrariness of the numinous powers. The motives to produce such utterly subversive postulates, overthrowing past ways of thinking, must have been important ones. But the fundamental question is: How did anyone ever get the idea that it is not angry, loving, punishing, or compassionate gods, ancestors, or demons who determine events, but rather absolute inherent laws, whose author is unknown? Appearances never seem to suggest the existence of laws. Whether in the family, the clan, or the state—it had always been a matter of personal relationships in which the emotions of anger, love, revenge, or sympathy were responsible for interpersonal actions. Why would this not be valid for the whole universe?

Besides, are the laws of nature really so evident that they are visible by themselves? Assume we knew nothing about such laws and were requested to rely only on our senses of sight, hearing, touch, and smell. Would nature become so transparent to us that the laws governing it would be recognizable? What inherent laws would be discernable to us through these senses, without any prior knowledge?

Let us take a look around. What we understand today to be the laws of nature, the inherent laws of physics and chemistry, has been taught to us in school, if not by our parents. When the natural sciences emerged two millennia ago in ancient China, it was initially a matter of recognizing any laws at all in nature—laws convincing and clear enough to prevail over the notion of events being influenced by gods, ancestors, and demons.

We could point out the simplest regularities. To start with, there is the succession of day and night. This is the most basic pattern noticeable to any attentive observer: each day is followed by a night; each night is followed again by a day. In an agrarian culture, the succession of the seasons is just as impressive in its regularity. There are regions in China where, in contrast to Europe, a succession of distinct seasons can be followed quite accurately to within about fourteen days. But what does that prove? Why should such occurrences lead to the assumption that there are laws explaining everything, controlling everything that happens in nature? For millennia, there was this alternation between day and night. For just as long, the steady sequence of the seasons determined the habits of sowing, cultivating, and harvesting field crops. For just as long, people noticed that objects fall downward, not the other way.

So why was China the place where people created a science in the third century BC? Why was it at this time that people in China doubted the influence of the numinous on events and claimed that inherent laws controlled everything past and present? It is unlikely that people's intelligence suddenly changed at that time. The inherent laws now postulated were just as recognizable or unrecognizable as they had always been. What event might have occurred to open people's eyes? What circumstances in 300 BC, against the backdrop of only the visible and eternally valid banalities of the alteration of day and night and the sequence of the seasons, might have led people at precisely that time to assume a linking of all phenomena and inherent laws pervading everything?

It is very astonishing that so many textbooks on the history of science so blithely ignore this volatile question, which touches on science's very understanding of itself. It also touches on medicine's understanding of itself, since medicine uses science for the endeavor to interpret the "normal" and "abnormal," healthy and sick processes in the body, and to derive instructions for action from such interpretations—instructions that should protect health and keep illness at a distance, or if illness has occurred, to heal it.

So let us ask ourselves what event might have occurred in 300 BC in China to open the eyes of first a few and then ever more people to the idea of a sweeping pattern in the events of the universe. Nature itself had not changed, nor had people's intelligence. Neither the observer nor the observed experienced any sort of change that would be grounds to recognize laws of nature.

4 | Longing for Order

The only thing in humankind's visible environment that is constantly changing is society—society in the sense of the entirety of the structures within which humans live together. Today, we are used to the fact that society changes fundamentally in a person's lifetime. As a child, a ninety-year-old person in Germany today might have seen the emperor. Certainly he or she will have witnessed the incredible changes in communication and technology, from the blackboard to the personal computer and from the horse and cart to the international space station. These and many other similarly breathtaking technical innovations are part of the social changes of the past century. We accept these changes and can hardly imagine the tranquil times when a long life could begin and end in the same era and society.

Despite constant change in history, the intensity of change has varied. The era in ancient China that saw inherent laws of nature being recognized and formulated lasted for a century or two. It was a turbulent era marked by far-reaching, radical change. At the end of this era, a very decisive event led to a completely new kind of social order. From these long-term changes, the Chinese laws of nature were developed; from this decisive event, a new medicine emerged. What happened?

In the eighth century BC, a political structure in China collapsed due to disputes over succession to the throne—a political system that, if the sources do not deceive us, had long supported a stable feudal system. From about 500 BC, many states of varying populations and sizes battled with increasing resoluteness for dominance. An ever smaller number of increasingly larger kingdoms fought on, changing alliances back and forth, for a long time. Eventually, in the third century BC, the ruler of one of the remaining states, Qin, won the struggle. In 221 BC, he achieved the first unification of China as a single empire under Qin rule. This centuries-long process was both traumatic and creative, particularly in the final three centuries, which historians call the Warring States period. Traumatic, because the changes destroyed the obsolete order. Creative, because they brought forth the foundations of the culture that we call Chinese today.

What relation did these processes have to the emergence of science? The discovery of inherent laws in nature falls in the final century prior to the unification of these kingdoms, and we may wonder whether this is a meaningless coincidence. Let us allow an authority on the social changes of the time—the only changes that took place—have a say. Sinologist Ralf Moritz of Leipzig has researched the fundamentals of Confucianism, the social philosophy advocated by Confucius and his contemporaries in reaction to generations-long turmoil and the maelstrom that threatened to devour all traditional structures. Confucianism, just one of many philosophical systems at the time, sought to guide the return to social harmony. The order they created in the end was admittedly completely different from what some of the social philosophers were hoping to restore.

> The ideas of Confucius (551–479 BC) ... are a reaction to cataclysmic turmoil in the wake of structural change in the old Chinese society. The world collapsed in which the intra-familial morality was simultaneously the state moral code. ... The Master responded with his therapy of world-healing, a reconstruction program targeting the "restoration of rites." ... The original meaning of rites is religious: rites as communication with the spiritual world, having the goals of attaining well-being and averting harm. Thus, thanks and intercessions gain ceremonial expression in the rites. ... As rites acquired the important function of regulating the relationship with ancestors, the transfer of ritual rules to the relationships between living family members, above all within the aristocratic elite, was an inherent consequence. ... [Rites] became the embodiment of correct behavior in the sense of the ... morality that had become conventional, while expressing socio-political structures.[1]

Thus, the world was put in order. Society included the living and the dead. Rites were the expression of communication between the living and their ancestors, but even more, they provided a basis for orderly human relations. It seemed to the philosophers that during the centuries-long war, when every man fought against his neighbor, communication and order had both failed. The philosophers strove for the image of the right path or "way" (dao) of behaving that people had strayed from. To the philosophers, the Way was the essence of order. Thus, following the Way would produce order—to Confucians, order in society; to Daoists, order in the universe. When the Way was lost, not only was order itself lost—the enduring wars had shown this all too clearly—but the vertical structures also broke down. Confucius, like the other philosophers of the era, saw that humanity must be guided anew in the right direction, leading to the Way, and with that, to order. As Ralf Moritz wrote:

> This suffering [of Confucius] due to disorder, and his resulting attempt to restore order in the world, forced the drafting of regulating strategies. ... Thus, Confucius' teachings form the first argumentative concept of people living together, the first produced in the history of China. ... In Lunyu [The Analects], rites appear as methods: children serve their parents, the living serve their ancestors; also as the guiding principle of politics ... respect for

others . . . abstinence from despotic power at the top . . . mirroring a new
kind of need for social order. Against this backdrop, a new ethic was developed, resting on the idea that the individual makes a conscious decision to
functionalize himself for the order of a greater structure, and sees himself
in this context. . . . The generalization of Confucius' order principle not only
required a general framework, but in addition proposed the realization of
this principle to always be the suitable response of a social subject to a concrete situation.[2]

A philosopher recognized the need for order. To change the plight
of the time, order was needed. He gave the term *dao* to this order. With
the image of the *dao*, the Way, he coined the term that would become the
foundation for Chinese ideas of order, for interpersonal relations just
as for all other events in the universe. The "cataclysmic turmoil" of the
Warring States period led Confucius to assume that healing could be
attained if man again saw himself to be part of a whole. The individual,
it follows from the teachings of Confucius, must be brought to realize
that his actions are meaningful for the well-being of the whole entity.

This is the first decisive point we need to grasp. An order exists, according to the new insight of Confucius and many of his contemporaries,
and this order does not consist of a random juxtaposition of countless details. This order can only be imagined using the realization that
every individual, because of his or her involvement with all others, has
a responsibility to contribute to the greater order through his or her
behavior.

5 | Ethics and Legality

It seems that this realization caught on. It did not stop with people; it
spread to the totality of everything. Was not the whole universe an edifice
of correlated and corresponding phenomena? The concept of systematic
correspondence, the foundation of Chinese science, was born. There is
no indication that what primarily impressed a person like Confucius
was the order of nature itself or an actual system of correspondences in
nature that later found entrance into the social philosophy. Rather, the

distinct opposites of order and disorder, harmony and chaos were only knowable from social reality, after looking back at centuries of human behavior. It was only after this knowledge had been attained that the simultaneous projection of the concepts of order and of systematic correspondence from society onto nature could occur.

This is the origin of the doctrines of yin-yang and the five agents. The latter was initially conceived of expressly—and the sources are very clear about this—to explain social and political change. Only in a second step was the doctrine of the five agents expanded to explain all kinds of change. Change is the temporary dominance of certain agents. This inspired the great Sinologist and physician Franz Hübotter to speak, at the start of the twentieth century, of a doctrine of five phases of change. Today, one generally speaks of the doctrine of the five agents. The yin-yang doctrine of the dualistic correlation of all phenomena seems to have avoided taking this initial detour through the explanation of social relationships. From its earliest appearance in historical sources, it has been applied to the totality of natural phenomena. We will examine these two doctrines in more detail when we consider the origins of Chinese medicine.

We can now explain why the foundations for Chinese natural sciences were laid by 300 BC; but, so far, we have no indication of how this led to the assumption of inherent laws.

Law is the opposite of arbitrariness, or the randomness of actions, in which the decisions to act in one way or another follow no schematic instructions; they could arise from either emotions or from considerations of the present moment. Law, on the other hand, obligates action to follow a certain pattern. Someone who steals can be sentenced as a thief in accordance with the law. Emotions toward the individual perpetrator should not play a role. A judge who lets emotions enter into his judgment departs from the law and acts arbitrarily.

Such arbitrariness is a characteristic feature of the usual behavior of people and also of the gods created in their image, indeed of the numinous powers in general. In human society, the arbitrariness of rulers can become a nightmare. In the family alliance or clan, in the small, manageable scope of daily interpersonal relationships, one can know

who likes or dislikes whom. Advantages or disadvantages conferred
upon one person from the attitudes or activities of another unavoidably
lead to affection or aversion. These feelings, in turn, result in certain
patterns of behavior. Since the origins and expression of affection or
aversion are known in the family or clan, there is a predictable pattern
of interpersonal behavior arising from such emotions. When behavior
unfolds that one would not have predicted, it is explainable, at least in
retrospect. Arbitrariness on this level is therefore foreseeable, and not
frightening.

If the ruler of a large political entity acts arbitrarily, it is a different
matter. The ruler is too distanced from his individual subjects for the
latter to be able to predict or know in retrospect what motives gave rise
to a particular arbitrary action. As long as the action is considered pleas-
ant, this can be overlooked. However, life for the subjects becomes a
nightmare when—and experience has shown this to be the rule—the
ruler's arbitrary actions intervene in a way that are felt to be unpleasant.
Military service, corvée, and tax burdens are examples of this.

Why this digression on law and arbitrariness? Chinese sources allow
us to look back into a time when the relationship of the rulers and the
ruled was still defined by an "intrafamilial moral code" that also served
as the state moral code.[3] The structures were still of manageable scope,
and arbitrary actions by the ruler were understood by the ruled in the
same way as arbitrary actions in the family or clan. With the emergence
of ever larger political units during the centuries of the Warring States,
the distance between rulers and subjects grew. The family remained
the ideal model for the state. But intrafamilial morality was no longer a
suitable foundation for the rule of increasingly complex state structures.
Governing growing numbers of people made it impossible for rulers to
deal with individual cases at their own discretion, as the head of a family
would. The schematization of interactions between rulers and ruled and
between the rulers among themselves was born.

Not all contemporary Chinese thinkers and philosophers were convinced that the schematization of actions and the accompanying estab-
lishment of governing structures was the best future course. We will
hear from the Daoists, who were vehemently opposed to this develop-

ment. In the end, those whose views corresponded to the new political circumstances prevailed, and their philosophies paved the way for the necessary schematization of human interactions in the new and increasingly complex structures of the state.

Reliable decisions are required for large state units to function. Such reliability is attainable only through commitment to laws, rules, and regularity. It is possible that this requirement opened some Chinese thinkers' eyes to the fundamental existence of regularities in nature and to the requirement to conform to this regularity for survival. It now seemed that obedience was not best directed toward an arbitrary ruler. Obedience should rather be an adaptation to the patterns that are the basis for the regularity of all existence. Traditional obedience to the ruler was supplemented by an obedience that the ruled has the good sense to bring to all existence.

Until now, happiness and survival were primarily dependent upon obedience to the ruler. Now a further precondition for well-being was added: integration into regularity, a life in harmony with the rules. Numerous written statements from the third to the first century BC offer evidence for social theorists' attempts to cope with the new circumstances. For example, Shen Dao (350–275 BC), an influential philosopher, recognized: "Presently, the Way [dao] of state leadership and the laws [fa] of the rulers are not influenced by regularity [chang]."[4]

The Chinese word fa probably originated in a military context, where it referred to the strategic rules troops followed to gain victory. During the Warring States period, the term was expanded to include the regularity of rule of an entire state.[5] It implies a pattern or system and law-abiding behavior, as well as the idea of law in the sense of penal law, the Latin lex. This is why the terms Legist or Legalist designate representatives of the ancient Chinese philosophical school that emphasized the society-building power of schematized behavior.

Schematic, impersonal, regulated—these were the new qualities of successful governance. It was a radical rupture. The new era no longer needed intrafamilial morality to double as state morality; it now needed an order based on laws and rules. Sociopolitical writings mostly written in the third century BC or later were united under the name of Guanzi (stated as seventh century BC). The author of the following quotation, like several other philosophers of the time, had lost his belief in the good in people. Laws, above all else, were to become the foundation of any fairly peaceful society: "From time immemorial, men have hated each other. The heart of man is cruel. This is why the ruler makes laws *[fa]*. From the application of the laws, rites arise. From the performance of rites, order grows."[6]

This certainty was united with the Confucians' ideas of order, as the schematization of behavior embraced Confucius's new morality anchored in the "restitution of rites," which was tailored to the complex state. The outline of a social philosophy had been developed, one that would prove to be a most suitable foundation for the united and highly complex empire that arose in 221 BC following the Warring States period.

Let us pause for a moment and consider the conditions surrounding the development of medicine in ancient China. Medicine is the linking of healing with science. Healing that lacks a scientific basis is not medicine in this sense. There had been healing in China since prehistoric times: sources reveal ancestor healing, demon healing, and pharmaceutics in premedical theory and practice. But the emergence of medicine required the development of science; that is, the idea that nature is governed by a regularity, in accordance with certain laws. These laws are not issued by men or gods. They are patterns that cannot be questioned and that always give rise to the same effect from the same cause. Postulating the existence of such rules and regularities, then determining their characteristic features, and finally understanding their specific effects on the health and sickness of the human body—these are the steps in the development of medicine in ancient China.

Xunzi (ca. 300–230 BC), a philosopher who contributed substantially to converting Confucius's philosophical ideas into practicable political teachings, did not believe in spirits, nor did he believe that humans could influence the course of nature. He writes: "The course of heaven/ nature *[tian]* follows a regularity. [This regularity] does not exist because of [the good ruler] Yao. And it is not lost because of [the bad ruler] Qie. He who conforms to this [regularity] to produce order will have good fortune. He who responds to this [regularity] by allowing disorder will have bad fortune."[7]

The change in the meaning of the Chinese term *tian* mirrored the new trend. Originally, the character *tian* referred to a higher ancestor, then to the ancestors' dwelling place. Later, the personal aspect was dropped, and the character took on a meaning that, though it is usually translated as "sky" or "heaven," is very close to "nature." As Masayuki Sato appropriately formulated: "The movement of the sky/heavens now became a metaphor for unchangingness and regularity."[8] It was now one's duty to conform to this regularity, initially as a ruler caring for the welfare of the state, and later as an individual caring for one's personal health.

Let us summarize what has been said so far. What reason is there to assume that the insight process could have gone the opposite way? What evidence is there that it was nature or the body itself that suggested the discovery of higher inherent laws? The development of science in ancient China can be attributed to two certainties: First, to the certainty of the linking and correlation of all things. Second, to the certainty of the necessity of regular, schematized relationships of all things among themselves. Both certainties grew out of the stark impressions that the fundamentally changed social structures had made on some Chinese philosophers, and in turn from the impressions that their teachings made on further thinkers. Now we can understand why it was just at that time that such ideas emerged.

6 | Why Here? Why Now?

Let us continue to reflect upon the conditions that secured the acceptance of this thinking. Indeed, this is the most important development in the history of ideas. In every era, innumerable ideas are expressed, like seeds sown in the field of cognitive dynamics. But most of them dry up right away. Some ideas experience a short growth period, some enjoy limited attention before declining. The historian asks: What conditions make the soil receptive? Why do some ideas fall on fertile soil, flourish rapidly, and become viable for survival, perhaps even for centuries? Other ideas, while they might be taken into the soil, seem to find no reception, and their "truth" that is closed to contemporaries may only be recognized many decades or even centuries later. We now turn to the history of ideas. What gives an idea its plausibility (since we shall not speak of reality here)?

The plausibility of the correspondence of all things, the plausibility of required order in all things, the plausibility of regularity, inherent laws, the schematic course of all things—this plausibility sprang from the sociopolitical reality: from there it illuminated nature and finally, as we will see, also the problem of sickness and health. Yet social interests can also make an idea appear plausible, and give it plausibility. Tracing back these interests is a difficult task that we won't attempt here. But a few remarks on this will nevertheless be included in the hope of offering clues for answering our persistent questions: Why is it here, why is it now, that an idea proves to be viable?

The belief in the regularity of society that suggests inherent laws in the order of nature has consequences. He who studies the laws of nature and recognizes them can take things into his own hands. He is no longer dependent on the supposed mediation services of those who position themselves between the gods and man. One can argue whether the gods themselves had to follow the laws. But there is no doubt that laws of nature weakened the power of the supposed mediators. This is one reason why many of the mediators—priests and theologians—found it hard to unreservedly sanction the developments of the sciences, particularly in medicine. People who can attribute an illness to natural causes, who know the laws of etiology and pathology and can derive appropriate prevention or a helpful measures from them, lose their fear of sickness as the gods' punishment for sin. This results in the mediators losing power, as they can no longer use the fear of illness as bait to lure people into following a certain godly morality.

Laws in society limit the arbitrariness of a ruler—*if* a social philosophy gains acceptance that sees the ruler as subject to the laws. Laws in nature limit the arbitrariness of the gods—*if* the worldview seeing the gods as subject to the laws prevails. We can see both tendencies in ancient Chinese social theory and religion. There were certainly voices that, in contrast to the Legalists, demanded the subordination of the ruler to the law. Chinese religion was, with the emergence of the natural sciences, markedly depersonalized and ritualized in a way that secured harmony among the people, but did not promote the worship of deities.

The success of Buddhism and the "survival" of many deities in local popular piety are not in conflict with this observation. Quite the reverse: the attraction of Buddhism, introduced in the first century AD from India (i.e., from a non-Chinese culture), clearly shows that the dominant world view in China basically had nothing to offer that could come to meet the desire of many people for a god the father or god the mother. The idea of the regularity of nature may therefore have also complied with political interests in the Warring States period and later. We will return to this point again, from another perspective.

The basic conditions for the emergence of medicine in China were thus fulfilled. Our attention is of course directed not primarily at China, but at the origins of medicine. Much closer to us than China is Greece, probably the first cradle of medicine. Should we not have begun our observation of events in ancient Greece, so as to progress chronologically and geographically to then turn our gaze to China? I have already mentioned the reason to first look afar: in ancient China, the emergence of first science and then medicine out of older healing happened in a time that is comparatively well documented; also, we have enough sources to be able to get a good idea of the social and philosophical preconditions, even for prehistoric times. For Greek antiquity, this is much more difficult.

7 | Thales' Trite Observation

"There can be no observation without assumptions." For quite a while now, this remark by the historian of medicine Thomas Rütten has been undisputed in the history of science.[9] As for the history of medicine, the remark is too seldom used as the basis for research on the history of ideas. This is perhaps unsurprising, because it is no simple undertaking. For ancient Greece, the preconditions that shaped observation and perhaps even made it possible—of the nature of the universe in general and of the individual body in particular—are practically lost in prehistoric obscurity. Though archeology and later, written sources reveal much about the early part of the first millennium BC in the Eastern Mediterranean region, the detailed knowledge that would be desirable for answering our question is almost completely absent.

In the Eastern Mediterranean, as in China, medicine emerged against the backdrop of a historically older healing. We know of this healing from the literature of Homer and Hesiod, to mention two examples. And as in China, medicine in the Eastern Mediterranean needed as a precondition science; that is, the idea that there are inherent laws independent of place, time, and person. It is completely beyond doubt that the development of such a science in ancient Greece preceded the development of medicine. In the same way, it is beyond doubt that, as in China, medicine in ancient Greece made use of scientific knowledge. But it is hard to explain why science developed in the first place and what stimulated individual thinkers to try to explain the course and changes of things rationally, without falling back on myth.

Let us take a look at the great historian of medicine Henry Sigerist's (1891–1957) comments on this problem. The historical figure commonly thought to be the first scientist is Thales of Miletus, who was active around 585 BC. Sigerist describes Miletus's position as a flourishing trade center in Asia Minor, which subjected it to many influences via the water route to the west and the land route to the east. Already having been exposed to such varied stimuli, Thales' travels took him to Egypt, where—as Sigerist quotes the ancient historian Herodotus—seeing the periodic floods and fertilization of the Nile valley prompted him to try to explain this phenomenon of nature.[10] That may be how it happened. But are we content with this explanation?

Is the origin of European and now world science really to be found in this banality, proclaimed anew in almost every history of medicine overview, that a man travels from Miletus to Egypt, sees the floods and fertilization (or perhaps even merely hears of them), and after some thought comes to the conclusion that all life has water as its basis, that water is the basis of all life? Inspired by this insight, further ideas followed at intervals of two decades: Anaximander, in 560 BC, did not believe Thales and brought *apeiron*, an indefinite substance, into the debate as the origin of all elements. In 546 BC, Anaximenes, in turn, did not believe Anaximander and brought air into the game instead of water and *apeiron*. Perhaps he had observed that someone whose mouth and nose are held closed dies faster than someone who is refused a drink of water.

The remarkable banality of Thales' statement is not reduced by the mention of the mysterious exchange between the East and West in Ionia. Countless men must have traveled from Miletus to Egypt. Toward its end, Miletus had an outpost in Egypt, near present-day Alexandria. We should at least ask: why Thales? Perhaps someone before him had noted that water is the basis of life while viewing the Nile or fishermen in some Mediterranean port. We can read similar things in the compilation attributed to the Chinese philosopher Guanzi. The unknown author of chapter 39 discusses in detail, in a section that was possibly written in the third century BC, why water is the "source material of all things."[11] Yet this was three centuries after Thales' remark and does not explain why it was Thales who, with his remark, founded the European history of science.

Now, Thales was certainly not just anyone. Aristotle (384–322 BC) called him one of the first Greek philosophers; enough of his writings have been handed down to show that he was an exceptional person. In Thales' works, historians of philosophy find the question "why?" which is also a question of "from where?" They credit Thales and other pre-Socratic philosophers with interest in revealing the origins and causes of existence—the search for primary matter. Astronomical, meteorological, and also mathematical knowledge are all ascribed to the inhabitants of Miletus and the Ionic milieu. That is all well and good, but it explains very little. We still want to know why the banal observation that "water is the basis of all life" never occurred to anyone before Thales, or, if someone else had already stated something similar, why the seed of this idea failed to fall on fertile ground and start the debate that took its course with Anaximander and Anaximenes. Some external cause must have made the ground fertile. What was the nature of this cause?

Heribert Illig, a historian of art, has proposed the fascinating and provocative thesis that three centuries in the Early Middle Ages, from about 610 to 910, are purely a calendar forgery of the High Middle Ages.[12]

If this view is true, then the writing of at least the main part of the book by Guanzi would fall in the sixth century BC, and the solution to the puzzle would be very simple: Guanzi's teachings found their way from East Asia to Asia Minor. Thales took it and set a debate going, the flames of which were possibly fanned for quite a while by contacts unknown to us between China and Ionia, until they finally unfolded a dynamic of their own with the familiar consequences. That would be nice. But the three centuries can't simply be erased from the parchments of the Early Middle Ages, and so we have to search further in the dark.

To the difficulties that present themselves in the answering of this question we must add the fact that the three aforementioned sages were active only in Ionia (Asia Minor), and not in what is today known as Greece, in Athens for example. Knowing this, should we still consider "Greece" to be the cradle of science? Perhaps we should search among the details of the political and social structures of Ionia for the impulses that would give us a glimpse of the background of a unique cultural process, one that led the historian Charlotte Schubert to make the statement: "The special achievement of Greek philosophy in the sixth and fifth centuries BC lies in the . . . continuous rationalization of the concept of nature . . . the highest aim was the study of the laws of nature and also their imitation in behavior as much as possible. From the observation of nature, a model of inherent laws resulted that was transferable to all fields."[13]

In the beginning was the study of the laws of nature. This is anything but a foregone conclusion, of course; some external cause must have awakened this interest in philosophers. But once this interest had been awakened, the observation of nature and the recognition of laws of nature led to the conclusion that man's illnesses, and also his health, are subject to the same inherent laws. This seems completely logical and consistent to us today. But we must take care: "us" is an overstatement. "A great number of people" would be better. We mustn't forget that since Greek antiquity there have always been people, some of them highly intelligent and well educated, who have remained unconvinced that the model of the laws of nature is transferable to all fields.

Once again we are led to the fundamental question: What impulse allows a certain idea, a certain worldview to fall on fertile ground for many thoughtful, intelligent, educated people? Why might the same idea not be accepted by others who are just as thoughtful, intelligent, and educated? This is what happened with the idea that the laws of nature sufficiently explain all processes in nature, including health and illness. Some people in antiquity vigorously pursued this idea; the development of medicine from about the fifth century BC was the consequence. Other people in antiquity did not follow this idea and instead clung to previous ideas about the omnipotence of the numinous powers.

Even today, in an era when the application of the laws of nature derived from science makes it possible to send airplanes into the air and build bridges that span bodies of water several miles wide, this second group of people remains unconvinced that the laws of nature are valid for all existence. To them, one or several gods rule over these laws. It seems as good an idea as ever to pray to this god or to the saints and to ask for help to survive an airplane flight or keep a bridge from collapsing.

The idea of the omnipotence of the numinous powers has never been scientifically disproven—neither by the early scientists in China nor by the scientists of Greek antiquity. Proving the nonexistence of the numinous powers is methodologically impossible. Moreover, through the millennia, countless examples of amazing rescues or apparent coincidences (that human judgment cannot accept as coincidence) have shown clearly enough that this idea is absolutely justifiable. So why do some people resist supporting this idea while others cling to tradition?

We do not know and are therefore in no position to explain why it was Thales of Miletus, then Anaximander, Anaximenes, and later Heraclites (of all people) and several others, rather than anyone else, who set out on the search for the foundation of all existence in the laws of nature. In contrast to the astonishingly similar development, only a few centuries later in China, of science based on the discovery of laws of nature, with Greece it is difficult to expose the political and cultural setting in Ionia in a way that plausibly presents a link between possible changes in this setting and the opening of the view to the laws of nature. Influences from Asia on the early philosophers cannot be ruled out. This makes the situation even more opaque.

But perhaps we can proceed in a different way. If we can't recognize the motives that prompted Thales of Miletus and his colleagues to ask their questions, then we can at least ask ourselves what milieu noticed these questions and the changing answers. Out of the blue and without being asked, a certain Thales of Miletus claims that water is the source of all life. Very nice. But who cares? And why should anyone care?

Looking back from the twenty-first century, we can indeed be grateful to Mr. Thales, since it seems he set a development going that today has us sending planes into the air and building bridges over straits. But his contemporaries were obviously unaware of the possibilities! Why should they have listened to him? They surely had enough worries in their daily life that it was of doubtful use to them to realize that water, an *apeiron*, or air is the substance holding the world together. At any rate, it seems it took about twenty years until the next philosopher, Anaximander, reacted to Thales' statement, and then another twenty years until Anaximenes entered the debate as the third participant. Thales may have had students or listeners who discussed his statement without contributing much to the emerging debate. This would have been left to Anaximander. And so it continued, until an ever larger number of philosophers and scientists ultimately built a canon of knowledge that unfolded its own dynamic of further development.

So let us try to forget that we live in the twenty-first century AD. Let us try to imagine what was so fascinating about the statements of the philosophers of the sixth and fifth century BC that they were heard and further developed. It could not have been the prospect of planes or bridges spanning kilometers.

8 | Polis, Law, and Self-determination

As in China, the key to understanding the processes in Greece, including Ionia, seems to lie in the term *law*. The laws of nature in China received attention and were attributed importance to the extent that sociopolitical changes replaced the old morality of individual relationships with the regularity of behavior governed by laws. No longer were the arbitrary emotional whims or naked self-interest of despots, be they human rulers or numinous powers, appropriate for the new state and social forms. Replacing the old arbitrariness was a lawfulness of interpersonal actions and of government.

All world views in Chinese antiquity that tried to show the escape from the centuries-long Warring States period were equally suited to reestablish the desired harmony: Confucianism, Daoism, the Mohists, the Legalists, the yin-yang doctrine, and others. The spiritual currents that eventually prevailed were not measurably superior to the others. They were simply the most suitable overall for imparting a foundation to the new state form. The idea of "law," of "schematized" behavior, of obedience to the rules played a major role in this worldview. Equally important was the morality, aiming for harmony, that had been lost for so many centuries and was then defined completely anew.

Do we find anything similar in Greek antiquity? The sociopolitical setting is possibly recognizable, with the idea of law in Greece being pushed into the foreground so much that the historian comes to the conclusion we have already quoted: "The highest aim was the study of the laws of nature and also their imitation in behavior as much as possible. From the observation of nature, a model of inherent laws resulted that was transferable to all fields."[14]

Let us read one of the most intimate connoisseurs of Greek culture, H. D. F. Kitto, formerly a professor of classical philology at the University of Bristol. His work *The Greeks: On the Reality of a Historical Model* includes numerous statements that are very revealing: "The Greeks did not doubt for a minute that the world is not capricious and arbitrary: it follows laws and can therefore be explained. Even Homer, who preceded all philosophy, thought so, since behind the gods (sometimes equated with them) stood the shadowlike power that Homer calls *Ananke*, 'necessity,' an order of things that not even the gods can break through."[15] And:

> The ruler of the Greeks was the law, a law every Greek was familiar with and expected fairness from. If he lived in a pronounced democracy, then he took his own due part in government. . . . Any arbitrary regime offended the Greeks deeply. But when he looked over to the . . . Kingdoms of the East, then he saw . . . the rule of an absolute king, who did not govern by

themis or by laws coming from the gods as the Greek monarchs did, but who governed solely by his own knowledge, and who felt no responsibility to the gods.[16]

Even in just these first two quotes from Kitto's *The Greeks*, we find practically all the key words that we are looking for. We learn that as early as monarchic times, the law of the gods was binding for earthly kings. The gods themselves even had to submit to a certain basic order. We are told further that "the Greeks" were also aware of an alternative: the rulers of Asia, who were considered gods even during their lifetimes and were constrained by no laws in their rule. The Ionians lived at the crossroads between Greek and Asian worldviews. Could it be that they were much more aware of these differences than the Greeks in the motherland? Might this direct confrontation with despotism and the arbitrariness of Asian regimes have fostered a subconscious impulse to promote inherent laws, indeed law per se in all fields of human existence?

The replacement of the kings with a city-state administered by the citizens, the *polis*, in Athens and other cities all the way to Ionia, was a further step toward the Greek ideal of *eleutheria*, which Kitto calls the "consciousness of the dignity of being human." This dignity was only attainable for a Greek of antiquity if he participated in the governing of the state and was not subjected to the arbitrariness of a ruler. The laws served to counteract such arbitrariness.

In China from the fifth to third century BC, there were a large number of small and minute political entities that were in constant conflict. These warring states increasingly annexed each other, so that they were eventually reduced to seven states, and then two, from which a single state finally emerged as the victor. As a result, in the year 221 BC, after lengthy and traumatic infighting, the Chinese kingdom was founded. In Greece, development progressed almost in the opposite direction. "In Crete," for example, "where Idomeneus ruled as the only king, we find over fifty more or less independent poleis, fifty small 'states' instead of one. But it is not so important that the kings have disappeared; the important thing is that no kingdom exists there at all now. And what is true for Crete is valid for Greece as a whole, or at least for those parts of Greece that played a noteworthy role in history. . . . They were all divided into an immense number of independent and autonomous political structures."[17]

The sociopolitical distinctiveness of these "independent and autonomous political structures," the poleis, is the key to understanding the high value attributed to inherent laws and self-determination in Greek antiquity. Only where there is a foundation of law can the citizen of the polis, in rational self-determination, conduct government business in his own interests. The rule of law in the city-state is simultaneously freedom from the arbitrariness of despots. The search for laws in nature is therefore simultaneously the search for freedom from the arbitrariness of the gods. The number of people who followed this new trend and completely denied the power of the gods may have been negligibly small. To suddenly oppose the power of the gods overnight might have even been suicidal. In such situations, new ideas do not directly confront the status quo, but instead look for an indirect sphere of activity where the longed-for structures are easier to establish than in the sociopolitical reality.

Only those who shared this longing for a new structuring of the sociopolitical reality—consciously or subconsciously—favored the new "order" that the natural philosophers demanded for the whole universe. The "idea that the microcosm of human life can be placed in relation to the macrocosm of the heavens or the universe" was not arrived at through the observation of the microcosm and macrocosm![18] The part visible to the individual is too small. The signs are too sparse to make such a comprehensive statement based solely on the validity of what is visible. The philosophers must have received their impulse from a manageable sphere of existence, and that sphere was their own sociopolitical reality—no other reality was available.

It was the political will to change very specific political structures, or to consolidate such structures where they had already been introduced but were possibly endangered, that directed people's view to the new order of nature while simultaneously formulating, as a demand, the unity of the natural macrocosm with the social microcosm. Only those who—consciously or subconsciously—shared this political will favored the new science. We must not lose sight of the fact that the immense potential of science is only known to us today. In the sixth, fifth, and fourth century, this potential was not even recognizable on the distant horizon. The will to political freedom and self-determination, not the promise of airplanes and bridges, directed people's view to the laws of nature.

Let us look at a few more quotations from Kitto's *The Greeks*, to be able to comprehensively assess the setting that the polis offered:

> The Greeks saw a moral and creative power in the sum of their laws, in the *nomoi* of their polis. They existed not only to provide justice in individual cases, but rather to make a mark on, and to sharpen justice per se. . . . And therefore Sparta was admired for its *eunomia*, for its "endowment with good laws," because through its laws and institutions it raised its citizens in unusual perfection to an ideal. . . . Sparta was praised because it had not changed its laws for many centuries.[19]

> The next event we hear about is the drafting of laws that were published in the year 621 BC under a certain Dracon. Up to that point, there had only been orally transmitted customary law that was guarded and administered by the noble class, the successors to the monarchy. Hesiod had already made vehement accusations against "princes who . . . make crooked decisions." . . . In any case, the transmitted law was codified and published in all its harshness. It at least provided some protection against arbitrary oppression. . . . We see the political connection: the transition from monarchy, to aristocratic rule, to the Attic democracy founded in 594 BC by the economic expert and poet/author Solon (ca. 640–561 BC), who was temporarily vested with dictatorial authority, as a gathering of all citizens later confirmed by Kleisthenes to be the "single and definitive lawmaker."[20]

It is important that we acknowledge the all-encompassing scope of the new tendency. The effect of social politics on the understanding of nature cannot be more than a weak presumption unless we are aware of the diverse cultural forms expressing the demand for new structures and for a new order. Here is an example: "Thus the mature polis became an instrument for Aeschylus through which the law was fulfilled without chaos breaking out, in that public and general justice replaced private vengeance."[21] It is not by chance that the poet Aeschylus (525–456 BC) is famous for his dramas. In a subtle yet highly impressive way, they express humankind's longing for liberation from the arbitrariness of the gods. Aeschylus did not deny the existence of the gods. However, by holding each individual accountable for his or her own behavior, he put individual responsibility in the foreground—thus his demand that people must shape their own fate. Law provided the framework for this shaping.

We could look for further clues that would reveal to us what prerequisites based on the assumption of overarching laws of nature were necessary for science to emerge. But perhaps what has been compiled here suffices to support our argument's most important point. In Greece, the certainty of living in an order has evidently existed since prehistoric times. Gods, rulers, and the ruled were subjected to this order. By the sixth century BC, in some central regions of Greece, the prevailing political tendency was to free oneself from the arbitrariness of the rulers, whether gods or earthly monarchs, and to subject all actions to laws that applied equally to everyone. The small political entity of the polis made the intermittent realization of these ideals possible—albeit with some setbacks and protracted struggles. The goals were to establish inherent rules of governing and individual responsibility for self-determination.

It may have been this tendency that created the preconditions and impulses for the new view of nature. Nature itself did not possess sufficient powers of expression. However, once the sociopolitical ideals and the orientation of the new worldview were projected onto nature, it became interpretable. There are many examples (some of which we will examine in detail as we discuss the history of medicine in China and Europe) of political ideals finding their first expression in the rather innocuous framework of healing before being propelled into concrete political programs. With respect to Greek antiquity, we had to first illuminate the setting that was conducive to the development of the sciences and that produced fertile ground for the statements of the philosophers of nature. We may recall the questions we asked at the outset: Why here? Why now?

9 | The Individual and the Whole

We have looked closely at ancient China and Greece, two different civilizations in the last millennium BC, because in both places science emerged, and science is the necessary precondition for the development of medicine out of a long-established healing. To reiterate an earlier point, the precondition for the emergence of science is the certainty of at least some people that all of nature follows an order, and that natural processes are regular and follow laws. The hypothesis is that this insight into nature cannot originate in nature itself, but must arise from impulses in a discernable arena of human existence: the arena of interpersonal activities, including the experience of ruling and being ruled.

It is noteworthy that in Chinese antiquity, the consciousness of the necessity of laws emerged against a completely different backdrop than in Greek antiquity. In China, the increasingly larger political entity eventually required a departure from the arbitrary rule based on personal relationships and emotions. Chapter 80 of the *Dao De Jing* depicts a political philosophy that proposes the ideal of the smallest possible community, a community that seeks no contact at all with the neighboring villages, even though they are close enough to be seen and heard. This political philosophy profoundly criticized the formulation of laws by men and therefore found no application in the government of the unified Chinese kingdom—though its supporters nevertheless maintained a vision that remained a formative influence on Chinese culture. In Greek antiquity, it seems, the ideal of a government guided by laws could be realized only in the smallest political units, the city-states of the polis, since this ideal also comprised the self-determination of every individual full citizen—an aspect that will again be important to us in understanding an especially remarkable difference between Chinese and Greek medicine.

We can already mention another difference here. As we have seen, the idea of "order" in early Chinese science was also essential to the expression of the idea of systematic correlation and correspondence of all phenomena. This idea was accompanied by the certainty, above all in the Confucian political philosophy, that the conquest of the "cataclysmic turmoil" could be achieved by humankind once it recognized itself to be part of a greater whole. The individual, according to the teachings of Confucius, must return to the recognition that his or her actions are meaningful for the welfare of the whole. The aspired-to order is not simply a juxtaposition of endless details. This order is only imaginable if the realization is grasped that every individual carries a responsibility to contribute to the greater order with his or her behavior.

In Greece, at least in sixth and fifth centuries, we find nothing similar. The first signs of a correlation can later be recognized in Greek medicine, but no one knows where the impulses originated. But neither Greek science (the understanding of order in nature) nor Greek medicine are marked by the idea of categories of systematic correlation and correspondence of all phenomena. Thales, Anaximander, Anaximenes, and Empedocles (495–435 BC) laid out the direction for this, initially emphasizing the division of phenomena into their basic raw materials, and later into their elements. In Greece, the broader perspective of phenomena—so decisive for Chinese science—remained of subordinated significance. In contrast to the situation in China, in Greece there was no persistent "cataclysmic turmoil" lasting several centuries to thrust the necessity of restoring unity of the country into the general consciousness and focus a view of the systematic correlation and correspondence of all phenomena. No other impulse that could have led to such a worldview is discernable either.

10 | Nonmedical Healing

Medicine is the transference of scientific ideas onto the organism. If we accept this definition—and we want to do this, at least in this book—then in real life there can be no purely medical healing. For two millennia, medical healing has been accompanied by nonmedical healing. This is unlikely to change in the future. Also, even after two millennia, the endeavor to scientifically explain illness is still far from being crowned with final success. Even now, in the twenty-first century, medicine cannot manage without nonmedical healing.

Nonmedical healing is unscientific healing. We use this term in reference to the vast number of conventions that, for whatever reasons, have found their way into the explanation and therapy of illness. What they have in common is that habit is the only reason for their practice. Thus the name "convention." The only justification for such unscientific "conventions" is that it is the way it has always been done, or that everyone does it a certain way. In modern orthopedics, for example, serious observers estimate that such conventions constitute about 95 percent of all interventions by physicians and physiotherapists. Nevertheless, many patients feel an improvement of their state of health after the application of such nonmedical therapies that are legitimated solely by convention.

But that is not the point here, and polemics is not our focus. We want to concentrate on the narrow definition of medicine, to understand its emergence and its later development as a part of healing. The ideals of university education are solely oriented toward the goal of medical healing, although a closer look reveals that many medically uncharted areas are supplemented by nonmedical healing—not only in the teaching of theoretical medicine, but also in its application at university hospitals.

Nonmedical healing has survived, on the one hand, as a kind of gap-filler for the areas where science could not yet take hold. On the other hand, nonmedical healing also survives independently, on equal footing with medicine. This second aspect is what will interest us most here. It is definitely not the case that the intelligent are enthusiastic about medicine while the unintelligent believe in nonmedical (scientifically unfounded) healing. A look at subscribers to the various facets of healing shows that intelligence is evenly distributed among them. So why do some people choose medicine and others nonmedical healing? What influences these decisions? This is what we want to find out.

As we examine the emergence and subsequent development of medicine, we must take a look at the older, nonmedical healing. We should ask ourselves whether it is merely the failures of medicine, the inability of medical healing to heal all episodes of physical and spiritual suffering, that has afforded nonmedical healing a niche for so long.

Now, many readers might be thinking: nonmedical healing doubtless has many positive effects. It doesn't matter that science has not explained every detail in the long chain of biochemical and biophysical events that account for the effects of leg compresses or quark compresses. These methods have their positive effects, and so they also have an unlimited future—at least as long as we do not become too forgetful in the course of being bombarded with advertisements for modern, commercial medicines. This thinking has validity. But we are going somewhere else with this discussion: we are dealing not with the level of effects, but with the level of interpretation.

Alongside state-of-the-art, scientifically based medical healing, there have always been alternative ideas of how illness arises, what the nature of illness is, and how to best prevent illness or find one's way out of ill-ness back to health. This is the level we want to examine. It is the level of theory, of worldview, and here is it reduced to ideas about the human organism and its components. So we want to find out, as we already have for the emergence of science: Why here? Why now? Why this? If we can answer these questions, we will know what medicine is. We will have gained knowledge that is of major consequence for health policy.

Let us turn to the two medical traditions that we can follow seamlessly from the present time back to their beginnings. The question arises, as it did in our discussion of the preconditions of science, to which should we turn first? To China and the roots of Chinese medicine? Or to the Eastern Mediterranean, where Greek medicine emerged on the periphery of ancient Greece?

For the same reasons we first discussed the origins of scientific think-ing in China, let us also begin our discussion with the origins and the early content of medical thought in Chinese antiquity. The availability of historical sources makes China much easier to study than Greek antiquity. We have excellent evidence of premedical healing in China. We can date China's early medical texts much more accurately than the early written sources of Greek medicine. And it was the examination of Chinese antiquity that was the impetus for this book. The situation in Greek antiquity, and also in all following centuries in Europe, is much more confused and muddled than the situation in China. Insights we acquired through our knowledge of the processes in China are what inspired us to ask the same questions about the European material.

11 | Mawangdui: Early Healing in China

Not long ago, the earth of China revealed a treasure it was entrusted with almost exactly two thousand years ago. This treasure is of utmost value for our discussion. In the year 167 BC, a noble family was buried in present-day Hunan province, near Changsha, the provincial capital. As was the custom in the upper classes of society, the dead were provided with all the important things of daily life for their "existence" in the afterworld. This consisted not only of maps, musical instruments, and many other things that were considered useful at the time, but also included a total of fourteen healing texts.

What a sensational find! The excavation in Mawangdui proved to be a direct probe into the cultural heart of the early Han era, only a few decades following the first unification of the Chinese kingdom in the year 221 BC. Since then, further graves of this era have been found and opened. They corroborate the impression left by the finds from Mawangdui. There was evidently an exchange of books across great distances. A network of authors, book collectors, and readers was in a geographical position to establish and maintain a market for literary products. In this manner, technical and philosophical texts found their way through the great kingdom. Here, of course, we are interested only in the texts on healing.

Let us assume that the texts such as the ones from Mawangdui were not written the day before his lordship's book collection was laid into his grave. They probably date from the late third to early second century. They tell us that intellectuals of the time saw the cause of illness mainly in two harmful influences. First, the harmful influence of a manifold host of spirits and demons, and second, of an equally varied host of microorganisms. To us, the idea of microorganisms seems like a good one. We would refer to microbes or even bacteria and viruses. Of course, we also think of worms that occasionally show up in orifices or in the stool. This is our reality.

This reality also existed in China, two millennia ago. Even today, at the beginning of the twenty-first century, worm infestation of the human body is so widespread in some regions of China that local residents assume a normal, healthy person must be infested with worms, as long as there aren't too many. It would indeed be harmful to have none at all in the stomach or belly. We need a few, otherwise digestion would not work. There are no objective standards for what is normal or what is healthy. The setting of norms and the accompanying demarcation of health and illness is always a cultural achievement.

As for the spirits and demons, we are tempted to say that such superstitions have existed everywhere at some point in the past. Is that really all? No, the belief in spirits and demons is not a thing of the past. Like the knowledge of microbes, viruses, and worms, it is part of the present. The terms may have changed. But in the West, large parts of the population believe in God or angels. To be more precise: they are certain of the existence of God or of angels. What makes them so certain? The fact is that for very many events, there is no explanation other than that it must be the work of God or of a guardian angel. Those who reject this explanation must do without any explanation at all. But most people desire an explanation for everything. And they wish for someone with superhuman abilities to stand above their day-to-day problems, reacting to urgent requests and prayers and putting things right. Countless examples corroborate such knowledge.

And so it was in China, two millennia ago. One lived in a world where spirits and demons existed, just like worms and other microorganisms. Microorganisms infested the grain, and it became "sick," died, decayed and was no longer edible. It seems obvious to assume that in leprosy, the most terrible scourge, the same microorganisms were at work. With leprosy there is visible decay from the inside out. Nose, cheeks, gums, fingers, and feet decay. And all this without a visible external cause. Evidently it was a worm making you rot away. The same worm that made the grain rot. This we read in the healing writings from the Mawangdui grave of 167 BC.

Worms or microorganisms were responsible for many illnesses. It is impossible now to say what particular thought processes led to some illnesses being attributed to the microorganisms while others were attributed to the effects of spirits and demons. Today, we say someone had a "stroke" because people in earlier times had the insight that the person must have been "struck" by something. Out of nowhere. That can only have been a certainly existent, but nevertheless invisible spirit. Just like lumbago, known in German as *Hexenschuß* (witch's shot). In former times, anyone could imagine how it would feel to be shot in the back with an arrow. That same feeling, but without any visible arrow or shot, could only be caused by an invisible enemy. The thought process in Chinese antiquity must have been similar.

Help was certainly available to counter the effects of the demons, spirits, and microorganisms. You could talk to demons and spirits. With apotropaic spells, people brandished their alliances with more powerful spiritual beings: Disappear, commanded the healer or the afflicted, or I'll get my ally and *he'll* show you! This often did the trick. Even today, anyone can try this out and might be surprised at the number of illnesses that can be effectively treated in this manner. Not all illnesses, of course. But enough to reinforce the certainty of the effects of spirits and demons.

Microorganisms could also be led astray from their destructive work, in manifold ways. You could not talk to them. But they could be chased out of the natural orifices. You could kill them if they stayed in the body. Vomiting and sweating were effective for removing the evil intruders. None of these ancient Chinese healing methods is theoretically or technically foreign to us today.

Knowledge of the appearance of the body's interior had similarly been maintained in writings on healing. There was a complete set of individual hose-like vessels in which something could move about calmly or excitedly. Blood, for example. Blood flowed out of wounds, and women lost it during childbirth and in monthly periods. Too much blood loss led to death. Who could dispute the essential function of this liquid? In addition, the mysterious qi moved in these hose-like vessels. No one had seen qi. But it was unquestionable that it existed and that it was essential. Qi moved through the mouth and nose, and in and out of other orifices. Closing the mouth and nose for even a few minutes resulted in death. Who could dispute the essential function of qi? There are no records of exactly what ancient observers imagined this qi to be. The character for qi, perhaps intentionally created to designate this new concept, depicts "steam rising from rice." Writings from the first century BC lead us to conclude that qi was thought of as a finely distributed, air-like material. It could condense and take visible form as solid material. It could also dissipate invisibly into the air.

The eleven hose-like vessels through which blood and qi rushed were palpable at different points of the body. The throbbing at these points varied in intensity. Some of the vessels were connected with an organ, such as the heart. But the vessels were not connected with each other. This was yet to come.

We could discuss much more about premedical healing and the image of the body in ancient China in the late third and second centuries BC. Nevertheless, what has been said here should be a sufficient basis for the discussion of the beginnings of medicine that later developed against this backdrop. Interested readers may refer to American Sinologist Donald Harper's translation of the complete writings found at Mawangdui.[22] Let us continue here by recalling that premedical healing in China was based on the idea that illness was caused by spirits and demons, worms, and other microorganisms. Treatment included magic spells and a remarkably rich pharmacy. The ancient Chinese pharmacy comprised over two hundred natural substances, mostly of plant origin, that, using painstaking procedures, could be transformed from a raw state into medicaments and from medicaments into dosage forms such as pills, powders, baths, and salves. In addition, a sophisticated vocabulary for the many technical procedures shows us the advanced state of the pharmacy of the time. It is certain that these drugs were at least as effective as magic spells.

This was the situation at the outset of the second century BC in China. Intelligent people and attentive observers of nature had arrived at varied insights into the regularities of nature and the causes of illness. They shared these insights across great distances in countless writings. They also applied these insights to healing the sick. They were as sure of themselves then as we are of ourselves today when we teach our present knowledge to students. Yet mere decades later, in the first century BC, healing in China took on a completely different form—medicine emerged for the first time. How did that happen? This is what we want to find out.

12 | Humans Are Biologically Identical across Cultures. So Why Not Medicine?

Healing becomes medicine when healers recognize laws of nature and seek explanations for the body's functions only with the help of these laws. We argued this at the outset. At first glance, it seems strange that different kinds of medicine have existed over the centuries in different cultures. How often have we heard that Western medicine and Chinese medicine are "alternatives," or that because of their different natures, they are "complementary" to each other! The truth of these statements will have to be discussed. For now, our questions are: What aspects are shared and what differences divide the two medical traditions in East and West? What continuities exist and what innovations divide the past and the present? Once we have answered these, we can ask: Where do the shared aspects and the differences come from in the two medical traditions of East and West? Where do the continuities and innovations come from in the comparison between the past and the present?

As for historical development and innovations, a first plausible answer could be that constant effort by researchers, naturalists, and clinically practicing physicians in direct contact with patients led to continuously better insights. This is the foundation of medical progress, which went hand in hand with technological progress. This cannot be dismissed. Pacemakers and artificial hip joints would be unthinkable without technological progress and the discovery of new materials. But for now, we cannot be sure whether this is also true for the founding assumptions of healing in general or the part of healing we call medicine.

A possible answer to our question about the source of differences between the medical traditions in the East and West is that such differences spring from religious and cultural distinctiveness. This sounds plausible, but it doesn't explain much. In fact, we will see that there is no representative medicine for "*the* Chinese culture." There is also no single representative medicine for the whole "European culture." There may be medical traditions that seem to dominate development, but that's about it. In China as in Europe, there have always been diverse groups subscribing to different ideas about the causes of illness and how to prevent or treat it.

We may confidently assume that the biological foundations of intelligence exist to the same extent in all civilizations. We may also assume that the biological foundations of illness and health are almost identical everywhere. Of course, there is evidence of minor differences, for example in the endowment of enzymes in various peoples that lead to variations in the tolerance of milk products or alcohol. But these minor differences are of little interest to us. The point is that a toothache is a toothache everywhere—even if the ability to deal with such pain, or to tolerate it, may vary.

There is evidence that members of some cultures attempt to "swallow" their pain. In such cultures, pain is an enemy that must never gain the upper hand. Pain is to be taken like a punch. In other cultures, it is common practice for people to communicate their pain to others and demand sympathy by wailing loudly.[23] Of course, such differences change nothing about the fact that pain is a cross-cultural and historically continuous aspect of human life. One could say the same thing about ulcers, nosebleeds, coughing, or malaria, to mention only a few examples.

So we have, on the one hand, humankind. We are an observer of ourselves and of our environment, nature. In every civilization, we are endowed with the same measure of insightfulness. On the other hand, we have the reality of the manifold conditions that, in all eras and across all cultural borders, are seen as illness, as undesirable, as deviations from the norm. So why do different images result when the reality is the same for everyone and the observers have the same intelligence? Apparently, there is something that pushes itself between observer and observed, something that is responsible for these differing images, both in intercultural comparison and in historical sequence. We want to reveal the filter that causes the same image to be seen in different ways. This filter determines the distinctiveness of the medicine of each culture and each era.

13 | The Yellow Thearch's Body Image

Let us return to Chinese antiquity. From historical documents, we can reconstruct the beginnings of medicine from the second and first centuries BC. Below, we will refer to these documents as the writings of the Yellow Thearch (also known as the Yellow Emperor), since it was under this name that they were handed down. There is a startling difference in content between the writings of the Yellow Thearch and the contents of the manuscripts excavated at Mawangdui. In the Mawangdui manuscripts, we read of eleven separate vessels partially connected with separate organs. In the writings of the Yellow Thearch, we find the description of highly complex systems of vessels in three different orders of magnitude.

First, there are the twelve great pathways. Three parallel vessels with four subdivisions each run from the torso to the fingers, from the hands to the head, from the head to the toes and from the feet back to the torso. These twelve sections comprise the twelve great pathways. They are interconnected and comprise a free-flowing system. Their contents, blood and qi, flow ceaselessly under normal circumstances. The body has two pathway systems: one in the left half of the body and one in the right half. There is no transfer from one half of the body to the other.

In addition to the great pathways are "network" vessels. These act as links between the separate sections of the great pathway system and together comprise a comprehensive network. A third level includes "grandchild" vessels. These depart from different places in the network and end somewhere in the tissues. (The description of further vessels, such as ones serving as reservoirs for eventual overflow if the great pathways are too full, can be omitted here.) The central idea is that the pathway system is made up of vessels of varying importance through which blood and qi flow to supply all body parts and organs.

Flow through these vessels is not simple unidirectional circulation. For example, different currents can meet in the same pathway. There are different proportions of blood and qi in a single segment of any vessel, although each vessel segment is seamlessly connected to the next. Congestion can result if an outside intruder enters a vessel. Examples of such intruders are dampness, cold, and wind. Whole regions can be cut off from the flow of blood and qi.

The writings of the Yellow Thearch paired every great pathway on the left and right sides of the body with a well-defined organ. In total, twelve organs stood in direct connection with the two pathway circuit systems. The organs themselves are described with astonishing precision. Ancient texts include descriptions of organ weight, position, size, and volume. In no way were the organs indiscriminately lined up, irrespective of their importance. Different organ hierarchies were suggested by various authors. One author convinced his fellows that lungs, heart, pericardium, spleen, liver, and kidney represent a group of organs. He called them the "internal depots." This Chinese term refers to the place where important things that one does not want to give away are stored. He called the small intestine, large intestine, stomach, gall bladder, bladder, and the so-called triple warmers "external depots." The Chinese term is used for places where things that are to be given away are stored.

Another author soon used the term external depot in a new sense: "official residence of the governor," or "palace." The author explains that each palace in the body is assigned to a "governor," who controls the "ruled." Thus, the liver, a "governor," resides in the gall bladder, a "palace," and is responsible for the well-being of tendons and membranes. The spleen resides in the "palace" of the stomach and is responsible for the muscles. The "palace" of the large intestine is subordinated to the "governor" lung; the lung governs the skin and hair.

Soon after this, yet another author propagated a new hierarchy. He identified the heart as the ruler, the lung as the chancellor, the spleen and the stomach as granary officials, the liver as the general, and so on. Each organ was assigned its position in the bureaucratic apparatus of the organism.

14 | The Birth of Chinese Medicine

It is now time to take a look at the medical laboratories and research facilities from which this knowledge may have arisen. What we have read in the preceding sections is a mere fraction of the knowledge that found entrance into the new medicine. So far, we have only hinted at the morphology and physiology of the new medicine. A completely innovative etiology (theory of the causation of illness) is also described in the writings of the Yellow Thearch. Demons and spirits are no longer considered at all. Neither are microorganisms. The focus is on environmental factors as the trigger of disease. We have already named some of these triggers, such as warmth, dryness, fire, heat, wind, cold, and dampness. These are triggers, but not the cause of disease.

The causal chain described in the ancient texts is not as primitive as one might expect of a system that was developed two millennia ago, far from all modern knowledge. Emotions are the source of illness. Passionate expressions of emotion weaken the organism, opening it to intruders from the environment. Cold, heat, wind, and dampness are basically natural companions to man in his environment. They cannot harm the organism when basically normal behavior is practiced. One should naturally dress warmly in winter and lightly in summer. However, environmental factors can play a role as triggers of illness when sadness, happiness, brooding, anger, or career worries cause an "emptiness," or breach, in the respective organs responsible for these emotions—a breach that allows environmental factors to invade. Here is an example: The heart is the refuge of happiness. He who expresses too much happiness deprives the heart of its contents. The fire of summer heat invades into the resulting emptiness and causes illness.

However, the body is not defenseless against these invaders. Day and night, various kinds of qi—referred to as the "military camp" and "protective forces"—patrol the surface and interior of the vessels. If the protective forces encounter invaders, a battle takes place, which the patient experiences as an attack of fever. If the protective forces win the battle, the invader will be destroyed. If the invader is too strong for the protective forces, it will find its way inside and will be in a position to interfere with all kinds of functions.

We could stop this account here or continue it for pages, or even several volumes. Evidently, the period from the second and first century BC to the third century AD was an extremely creative phase, when many new ideas flowed into medicine. Let us look at one last point, the treatment of illness. The creators of the new medicine took pains to emphasize the value of prevention. As one of the authors put it, you do not wait until you get thirsty to dig a well, and you do not start forging weapons in the middle of a battle. So why only start treating illness when it has already broken out? Consequently, the new medicine offered many instructions on how to avoid the dangers of such harmful climatic factors as wind and cold, on learning to control one's feelings, and much more.

But as experience has shown us time and again, illness is nevertheless reality. The new medicine looked at dietary strategies for prevention and therapy. The focus, however, was on two other procedures. One of these was bloodletting, the other was the pinprick. Bloodletting was an ancient therapeutic technique for removing quite a few of the invaders splashing about in the blood in the organism's vessels. However, a milder form of therapy increasingly emerged into the foreground: needle treatment. When it started in the first century BC, this needle treatment was not at all similar to what we now call acupuncture. The fine needles in use today did not exist back then.

In fact, we do not really know what instruments the term *needle* designated. There is a list that contains descriptions of nine different needles from the first or second century AD. These needles are nothing other than miniature weapons: mini-daggers, mini-swords, mini-lancets. They had round or pointed heads. But none of them bear any resemblance to today's needles. Today's debates on the precision quality of acupuncture needles and on how deeply to insert them—one millimeter, two millimeters, four millimeters, or more—for the best effects, are far removed from the crude instruments often mentioned in the same breath as "sharpened stones" in ancient texts. However the needles might have looked, they were in any case used to let blood and qi out of the vessels and to influence the flow of blood and qi in the body. They were supposedly capable of removing congestion, of correcting currents flowing in the wrong direction, and quite a bit more.

This convinced some intellectuals to consider such views useful, to develop them further, and also to apply them in the treatment of the sick. Medicine was born. Mention of the numinous powers of the spirits, demons, and ancestors had disappeared. Through the science of systematic correspondences, the human organism was submitted to the greater perspective of the laws of nature. From now on, the yin-yang and five agents doctrines were to be as valid in the body as they were in the distant universe. They aligned humans into a higher scheme of events, and they brought the promise of survival without illness through adaptation to this scheme of events.

The three or four centuries following the unification of China in 221 BC were a very dynamic time for human thought, even two millennia in retrospect. The new body image was applied to the explanation of all known illnesses. Whether it was the disease we call malaria, which differs so conspicuously from other illnesses because of the periodicity of its fever attacks and shivering fits, or whether it was a cough, back pain, or hair loss—all these and many other illnesses required a scientific interpretation. Even the question as to why body parts should be covered in winter while the face endures wind and weather caused quite a stir.

The scientists of the time found the explanations they desired in the teachings of systematic correspondences, coupled with the morphological knowledge gained by the act of looking at the body. They had logical ideas about why intermittent fever occurred in a rhythm of two, three, or four days. They knew the precise reasons as to why a cough developed in summer, autumn, winter, or spring, and even the cause of hair loss was not too much for them to explain.

15 | The Division of the Elite

It must have been an exciting time—a radical breakthrough into a new knowledge. From the perspective of those who participated, this might be an accurate description. But if we look closer, we see that only a very small part of the population was involved in this breakthrough. For the vast majority of the population—perhaps 70 to 80 percent, or even 90 percent—this new medicine was meaningless. And this would not change in the following two millennia. The knowledge and application of this medicine remained confined to a small elite up until its decline in the twentieth century. But we must qualify even this statement, since then, as now, it was not the entire elite of ancient China, or of the Han dynasty (206 BC–AD 220), that started and supported this development. In fact, the majority of the elite did not accept this medicine at all.

This makes one sit up and take notice. Why did the emergence of the new knowledge appear to some elites to be a breakthrough out of darkness, while others resisted the new knowledge, wanting nothing to do with it? Both groups were highly educated and literate. Both groups were familiar with the classical philosophers of the past and lived in a culture that we can justifiably call Chinese, even in those early centuries. What different filters stood between the observed and the observers, so that despite seeing the same object—nature and the healthy or sick person—they developed completely different views?

It cannot have been due to the expressive power of the body that some people set their course for the new medicine while others saw no reason to do so. Everyone agreed that fever was the heating of the body. Everyone knew that a nosebleed was the flow of red fluid out of the nose. Everyone considered an ulcer to be an unpleasant destruction of the skin's surface. We could list very many such expressions of changes in the body. In the end, however, it would only corroborate the impression that was already given by these few examples. The body can give the observer countless signs that there has been a change from a normal condition to an abnormal, sick condition. Yet the body cannot communicate the causes for this change or the processes occurring invisibly inside the body.

That's how it was in antiquity, when technical media were still quite limited. All body processes had to be visible from the outside: by looking at color changes of the skin or tongue, by smelling odors of the body or mouth, by listening to the pitch of the voice, or by feeling the pulse. Only the patient had a certain opportunity to "look inside himself." He could communicate his feelings spontaneously or at the request of an observer. It is not much different even today, despite our rich technical possibilities. Medical imaging lets us observe the live functioning of a heart valve, on a monitor. We can accurately depict details of cell division and many other processes. But even today, the most fundamental level of the causality of many changes remains hidden from view.

16 | A View to the Visible, and Opinions on the Invisible

Today, as in antiquity, the expressive power of the human body is limited to outward appearances. It makes only a fraction of difference that technological progress now allows us to see these outward appearances on the level of molecular biology. In spite of the limitations, observers in antiquity drew their conclusions. They described not only what is visible to the naked eye but also presented their views on what cannot be seen. Medicine survives on such views of the invisible.

Medicine is the linking of knowledge of the visible with knowledge of the invisible. By the visible, we mean the morphological structures of the body. These are, first of all, the gross structures that are perceptible to the naked eye. The head, nose, belly, and legs are examples of gross structures that are outwardly visible. Furthermore, there are the gross structures that can be seen only if the body is opened, such as the lung, stomach, and heart. Certain minute structures are also visible, such as the structures of individual cells. But to see these, highly developed technology such as an electron microscope is needed.

Included in the visible are also the body's changing colors and, in the figurative sense, changes in body temperature from coldness to warmth and vice versa, and the different smells of the body. In contrast, the invisible includes the laws that the expressions of nature on the higher level, and of the body on the lower level, are based on. Also included in the invisible are the links that exist in the body between separate body parts and the recognizable functions. A creator of medicine is an observer who integrates the view of the visible with his ideas about the invisible and draws conclusions from this about how to understand, prevent, or heal illness.

With that, we come a bit closer to the central point of our question. We want to know how the ideas of the invisible are formed. Turning once again to the beginnings of medicine in China, we can ask why some members of the elite of the time developed certain ideas about the invisible. Once we have settled that, we will understand why these ideas about the invisible seemed so unconvincing to other members of the elite. But what did these ideas about the invisible develop from? Uncovering the impulse for this will reveal a pattern that will make the whole history of medicine understandable—not only in antiquity, but in the course of the following two millennia. And not only in distant China, but also in our own European tradition.

The morphology of ancient Chinese medicine is of marginal concern to us here. We have already determined that some authors evidently had precise ideas about the physical dimensions of the body's major organs. The sources of such knowledge are obscure; records from the first century AD describe an intentional examination of the interiors of dissected corpses. But our interest lies elsewhere. The focus of our considerations is the transition from knowledge of the existence of eleven separate vessels in the body, some of which are paired with an organ, to knowledge of the existence of twelve pathways, each linked with a certain organ and comprising an integrated network of pathways. This idea does not come from the dissection of a corpse or follow from a visit to the butcher's shop. It is equally unlikely that these would give one the idea that there is an uninterrupted flow of blood and qi flowing through the body's vessels.

Similarly, the body's powers of expression cannot have been sufficient to inspire the idea of patrolling "security forces" through the skin and vessels, always on the lookout for invaders. How could anyone arrive at such insights by looking at a living or dead body? And even if we assume that the Chinese observers of the time had almost clairvoyant powers, the question still remains as to why these clairvoyant powers of the second or first century BC did not bear fruit a couple of centuries earlier. At any rate, nothing indicates that there was any sudden advance in people's intelligence.

The observational powers of the observers did not change in the sense that they were suddenly able to see something they could not see before. Nor did the thing being observed (i.e., the human organism) change to the extent that it suddenly revealed an integrated pathway network or protective troops.

The only thing that changed—and it changed profoundly—was the sociopolitical and national economic situation. Is this the key to understanding the new medicine?

17 | State Concept and Body Image

The year 221 BC saw the end of a centuries-long conflict between an originally large number of kingdoms that were eventually incorporated into seven, then five, and then three competing states. Finally, the ruler of Qin conquered his opponents and was able, for the first time ever, to rule over a unified China. From that time on, he called himself the "First Emperor of Qin." Following his victory, he was left with the job of making unity a reality. In the few years before his death in 204 BC, he was able to create an integrated whole out of states that for the most part had been culturally and economically independent. He ordered a common script, common track width (on roads), and common weights and measures, thereby laying the foundation for a lasting exchange of goods and people in his kingdom. This exchange was necessary to support the huge new cities in distant parts of the country. It was also necessary to administer the country with an increasingly complicated bureaucracy.

The new state organism offered China an experience it had never known before. It was the experience of being an organism consisting of several units, where each unit contributed to the well-being of the whole. All units were connected by a network of roads. Only if the traffic on these roads ran smoothly, if a person could travel without hindrance and transport goods from one place to another, was this state organism in order. This was something completely new. For some philosophers of the time, the effect of this new economic and social organism on their worldview was so profound that they could not avoid internalizing the model as a whole, extending it even to their understanding of the body.

Thus, the body organism in the new medicine was nothing but the state organism transferred onto the body. The various ideas that authors of the time recorded about organ function did not originate in the body's powers of expression. They originated in the reality of the new state. Now we can understand why an author suddenly had the idea that the body organism is an integrated collaboration of five governors who govern their respective subjects from their palaces and are linked among themselves by manifold paths, creating a greater whole through their exchanges.

The human organism, the observers and creators of the new medicine realized, rested on the same structures as the organism of the unified state. The word they used for "healing" was therefore the same word that was already used for "governing": "ordering" (zhi). They considered "illness" (bing) of the human organism to be the same as the "chaos" or "social unrest" *(luan)* of the state organism. The wise ruler, they wrote, does not heal illness but regulates the human organism so that no illness will develop. The wise ruler does not bring order to social unrest but governs the state organism so that no social unrest will arise.

18 | Farewell to Demons and Spirits

It would be too much to examine all the details of the new medicine, looking for parallels with the new structures in the sociopolitical and economic setting of the time. Below, we will focus on three things: First, the disappearance of demons and microorganisms from teachings on the causation of illnesses. Second, the understanding of the pharmaceutical tradition. Third, the question of the body's powers of self-healing.

Why did the demons and microorganisms disappear? Well, it is relatively easy for us to understand that the scientists of the time ignored demons. After all, most of today's scientists aren't very keen on speaking about demons either. So the existence of demons is simply denied. However, we mustn't forget that even for many of today's scientists, gods and angels are a tangible reality. So perhaps it is not so easy to understand why a part of the Chinese educated elite in the second and first centuries BC suddenly stopped believing in demons and the other spirits. What evidence to the contrary must have existed to prompt the sudden rejection of this knowledge, which had been passed down for centuries and was often very useful—including in healing illness through exorcism?

Demons and spirits are invisible to most observers. This would be one argument. Only that which is visible exists. But what about the microorganisms? They are visible to everyone. They creep out of orifices in the living and out of wounds in the dead. They are found in stool, and sometimes one even vomits worms that mistakenly took the way up instead of down. Why did these creatures have to forfeit their existence in the new medicine? Why did everyone stop paying attention to them?

Everyone? That would be saying too much. Not all scientists and observers were prepared to renounce the knowledge of demons. It was only those observers responsible for the new medicine who no longer saw what their predecessors had seen for many centuries. It was only in the new medicine that this old knowledge no longer had a place. However, in the pharmacy that dated from premedical times and accompanied medicine from then on as an alternative therapy form, the knowledge of the demons that are responsible for so many illnesses survived. What did the spirits and microorganisms have in common that caused the creators of the new medicine to ignore them while the advocates of pharmacy continued the battle against these pathogens?

This is a fascinating question. The "upper class of ancient China," literate and formally educated in history, philosophy, and natural history, is divided into two groups: one group comprising those who no longer perceived part of what was once reality (namely spirits and microorganisms), the other group comprising those who continued to acknowledge that part of reality and included it in their healing. What separated the two groups? It cannot have been biological intelligence, and it also cannot have been any characteristics of the observed. These things, and this can hardly be emphasized enough, were identical for both groups.

Let us venture to a higher level of abstraction to ponder what was happening in China at the time. What did the demons, spirits, and microorganisms have in common? Those who perceived them at all perceived them as enemies. They threatened the health and the life of humans. How did one deal with enemies? After an era of wars lasting centuries, people at the time knew that in war, friendly persuasion is not useful. In war, the only effective strategy is to threaten the opponent with retaliation or destruction before the attack. And to kill or banish the opponent who attacks anyway. This is how one also dealt with the demons and microorganisms. Prevention and therapy were organized as in war.

Demons and spirits were shown amulets or confronted with spoken exorcisms describing one's alliance with the superpowers of the numinous world, such as the sun, moon, Big Dipper, or especially fierce demons whose alliance one sought against the weaker spirits. If a demon had settled in the body, it was commanded to disappear; otherwise, there were ways to destroy it. Similar techniques applied to the microorganisms. However, microorganisms did not react to words, but, with the help of medicine, were either killed on the spot or chased out of the body by means of vomiting, purging, or induced sweating. What was it in this attitude toward the demons and microorganisms that seemed natural to the one group in the ancient Chinese upper class, but not to the other?

A closer inspection of the basic ideas of the new medicine reveals that they served the worldview of many, but not all, political groups in the early Chinese empire. The first group comprised those who were subconsciously guided by the necessity for lawful behavior in an increasingly complicated society. They also recognized inherent laws for all other areas of human existence and for all of nature. We are familiar with the implications that these associations have for recognizing the existence of laws of nature. In the new medicine, these laws of nature were now transferred to the interpretation of the human organism's functions. The relationships of the organs on different levels, among themselves, and with the course of nature, were now set on the foundation of the same regularity that was believed to have been already recognized in the order of social and natural processes.

A second political group had different motivations to participate in the development of the new medicine. They were not totally convinced that the new, complex state could achieve lasting harmony—superseding the centuries of chaos—solely with punitive laws. They missed the appeal to morality. Ethics and rites, they taught, should enter into everyone's flesh and blood. Peace and harmony can prevail only if everyone behaves in accordance with rank and position, as the ethics dictate. Morality must be renewed as the basis of human coexistence. Everyone who follows morality and ethics can expect a long, fulfilled life.

How do we see these ideas reflected in the new medicine? The inherent laws are easy to recognize. The yin-yang doctrine and the doctrine of the five agents account for all knowledge of the causality and characteristics of illnesses. Whether for back pain, hair loss, malaria, or a cough, in an exceedingly creative and dynamic process, countless scientists sat down and came up with explanations for all kinds of illness conditions. It was as exciting as the first consistent application of the biological and physical sciences to disease etiology and physiology in Europe in the nineteenth and twentieth centuries. One physiological process or illness after the next became understandable through the new science.

Exactly the same thing happened from 200 BC to AD 200 in China. A very exciting time—a point of departure. The success of this departure convinced scientists of the comprehensive validity of their laws of nature. He who lived in accordance with the state laws could live a peaceful life, free of punishment. This was guaranteed by the ruler and his bureaucracy. He who lived in accordance with the laws of nature could enjoy his allocated sphere of existence to the fullest: from birth through youth and adulthood, and on to weakening and death. Was not all life, in the state and in the universe, subject to inherent laws?

19 | New Pathogens, and Morality

Why did demons and the microorganisms have no place in the new medicine? What were the pathogens in the new medicine, if not demons and microorganisms? The new pathogens were not actually so new after all, but from then on, they were the only pathogens. Cold, dampness, wind, heat, dryness, immoderation or excesses in eating and drinking— these were the new "enemies." One referred to them with the comprehensive term *evil*. Evil is that which invades places it does not belong. Was that not also true for demons and microorganisms? If we for the moment ignore the "stomach worm" necessary for digestion, they were not exactly welcome guests in human bodies either.

There is a profound difference between the demons and microorganisms on the one hand and cold, dampness, and so on on the other. Demons and microorganisms did not fit into the new age of morality. They did not follow morality, but were outsiders to it. Demons and microorganisms had found their way into premedical healing at a time when centuries-long wars had damaged faith in morality and in the suggestibility of behavior through the appeal to good ethics. Demons and microorganisms attacked the same way invaders attacked—irrespective of their victim's behavior. Anyone at all could be a victim. They were fundamentally evil.

A new perspective was introduced here in terms of cold, dampness, wind, heat, dryness, and immoderation in eating and drinking.

These pathogens behaved in accordance with morality. Every person who ordered his behavior ethically and adapted himself to the laws of nature could assume that he would not fall victim to them. The certainty that these pathogens could be influenced by one's own behavior made it seem worth the effort of living in accordance with morality and ethics.

This was not always convenient. Who is not occasionally tempted to ignore good ethics? Only the promise of a great reward for the strict adherence to good ethics could bring about the sudden change from an immoral to a morally strict age. This reward had a dual nature: respect in society (social survival) and protection of health (physical survival). No room for demons and microorganisms here. They endangered the new goal. If people harbored the idea that it doesn't matter how one behaves—since virtuous and bad people get equally sick, or because pathogens are fundamentally evil and can't be tamed by moral behavior or agreements—then one of the most important motivations to follow the strict ethical code is lost.

We must not imagine that a commission or "expert council for medicine" sat down together and decided that from now on, demons and the microorganisms may no longer exist, because they endanger the enforcement of our moral program! This is certainly not what happened. Certain thinkers argued profusely against the abolition of the belief in demons. They basically suggested that fearing the spirits promoted ethical behavior. But the new medicine followed a different guideline. The existence of demons and microorganisms did not fit into the new understanding of the world. What sort of friendly persuasion or ethical behavior could keep a demon or worm at bay?

A second aspect was then added that negated the basis for the existence of these old pathogens. In the new medicine, the doctrine of the causation of illness and of normal functions in the organism was based on the idea of vessels linking all body areas and organs with each other. These vessels comprised a very complex pathway network for the transport of blood and qi, but things did not move through the network at random. Where, when, and how much the various substances moved was governed by very specific inherent laws—within the framework of systematic correspondences. Demons and microorganisms did not conform to this system of correspondences.

Was there any indication that in summer, autumn, winter, or spring, demons adapted to the seasons? With animals this could be assumed. Animals with feathers, scales, or fur behaved differently, in accordance with the seasons and thus fit into the system of correspondences. But the demons and worms responsible for sickness, generally invisible to the naked eye, were not part of this world. There was no evidence that these pathogens followed the laws of transport pathways in the body, so they could not be found in any certain place at any certain time. In contrast, cold, dampness, wind, and heat behaved in accordance with the laws of the system.

One last point was in favor of these new pathogens. The harm caused by cold, dampness, wind, heat, dryness, and immoderation in eating and drinking was reversible and could be healed. These pathogens did not necessarily lead to a lasting loss of health or to death. The new medicine recommended a variety of behavioral changes to get back on the right track, to remove these pathogens from the organism, or to correct the consequences of immoderation in eating and drinking. The new medicine promised full recovery for the repentant sinner.

One might behave wrongly, allowing cold or heat to invade the body. One might repeatedly fail to resist the temptation of delicious food and drink. The new medicine promised opportunities to return to the path of the law and that those taking these opportunities would be totally healed. The possibility of this "return to spring," as the beautiful Chinese metaphor of recovery goes, did not exist for harm that had been caused by microorganisms. Who had ever seen a leprosy patient's physical disfigurement disappear?

Do we now understand why the old pathogens no longer turned up in the new medicine? The political will to find a way back to a society guided by ethics and morality led to a new worldview, without the parts of the old worldview that were opposed to the new goal. Yet the new thinking contained yet another aspect that lets us understand why the old enemies no longer seemed to be in keeping with the times.

The new morality was the morality of moderation. Moderation in all things is not unknown to Westerners. Even in ancient Greece we find the exhortation, "Don't overdo it!" This was precisely the new morality in ancient China as well. It was applied to eating, drinking, and sex. It also expressed itself in the control of emotions. For a peaceful and harmonious coexistence of different people in a crowded area, few things are as harmful as the uninhibited expression of emotions. So the idea was to avoid giving free rein to one's feelings. Restraining emotions as much as possible was considered a necessary precondition for a peaceful society and also for a healthy life.

In the new medicine, this thinking was demonstrated in the certainty that happiness, sadness, anger, brooding, and worry are each linked with an organ. Immoderate expressions of these feelings lead to damage to the respective organ. Each expression of feelings costs the matching organ some of its strength. However, if an organ has already been weakened through immoderate expression of feelings, emptiness can arise there. An outside invader then enters the void. Here is an example: Happiness is produced in the heart. Too much happiness depletes the heart of its resources and weakens it. The heart then becomes vulnerable to the pathogen heat. Those who control their happiness do not need to fear being struck by heat. Demons and microorganisms did not comply with this system. From then on, they were ignored in Chinese medical ideas about the causation of illness.

20 | Medicine without Pharmaceutics

Demons and microorganisms were not the only things to be barred entrance to the world of ideas of the new medicine. Another hitherto well-trusted aspect of therapeutics was also excluded: the entirety of pharmaceutics. This is surprising! Imagine a historian in the distant future writing the following: "In the nineteenth century, modern Western medicine came into being. At that time, all normal and sick processes in the body were researched using chemical and physical methods and explained in detail. Pharmaceutics were initially left out! It was not until the twenty-ninth century that the characteristic features of medications and their effects on the organism were also explained with chemistry and physics, biochemistry and biophysics." Absurd? Indeed. We know how it really happened. Yet in Chinese antiquity, the transfer of the new science to therapeutics happened in the same way that we just imagined as an absurd hoax for Europe. The doctrines of systematic correspondence, yin-yang, and the five agents were used to explain only the normal and sick processes in the body. Medications and their effects were ignored.

How could this be? The writings from the Mawangdui tomb portray a very sophisticated pharmacy: the number of substances used, the variety of processing techniques for different dosage forms, and the spectrum of indications recorded in the manuscripts all document the advanced status of pharmaceutics. In addition, even in the present day, pharmacy is the backbone of traditional Chinese therapeutics. So why did it not find acceptance in the new medicine? This is a process even more exciting than the "losing sight" of demons and microorganisms.

We now know that only part of the educated elite of ancient China created the new medicine, turning away from demons, microorganisms, and pharmacy. We also know that another part of the educated elite did not participate in the development of a new medicine, and continued pharmacy as independent therapeutics—including the battle against demons and microorganisms. How did it happen that such a rift opened up—a rift that split the elite of ancient China? What filter positioned itself between the eyes of the observers of nature and humans on one side, and the observed on the other side, so that such different world-views could develop?

A view of the world always contains a conception of what is normal and what is abnormal, a crisis. Different worldviews are largely in agreement about this conception. Most people wish for freedom and harmony as the foundation for a fulfilled life. Different worldviews and sociologies exist because the recipes for attaining this freedom and the means for preserving this harmony vary greatly from one worldview to another. We are experiencing this in our own era, and it was no different in China two millennia ago.

In ancient China, political philosophers' opinions were similarly divided on the question of which path was the right one for structuring a peaceful and harmonious future. The social facts were highly visible: At first, ever larger kingdoms battled among themselves for dominance. A united Chinese empire was then created in the year 221 BC. The first emperor's administrative achievement, extremely impressive even from today's perspective, was the creation of a highly complex, integrated state from hitherto diverse individual states. In the decades and centuries following the unification of the empire, bureaucratic structures were consolidated.

So far, so good. The history of the Chinese empire following unification is a fascinating cultural legacy of power, recurrent ascendance and decline, art, poetry, and technological civilization. And yet there were always skeptics. In this kind of society, skeptics saw the roots of incessant conflict and social catastrophe. They opposed the idea of the harmonizing power of laws. The opposite was true, they argued. On the one hand, the constraints of laws on life were the true cause of much inappropriate behavior. On the other hand, the skeptics opposed the complex state as a suitable form of organization of human society, because they found it to be in total opposition to the way they believed society should be organized—in small, local communities. Each community self-sufficient and free of the need to engage in exchanges with a neighboring community. No trade with neighboring communities, and of course no military to pursue any expansions. Writing was also superfluous. A few knots tied in a piece of rope were sufficient to remember the past.

These skeptics of the suitability of the complex, unified empire—with its manifold trade involvements in widespread parts of the country, and its all-penetrating bureaucracy—could not endorse the new medicine. They possessed a different worldview. In this worldview, there were no laws, either manmade or natural. The processes of nature, the rules determining the course of nature, lay outside of human powers of imagination. Of this, the Daoists were certain. Any attempt to capture these rules in words, to explain them with human terms, would fail. Let us recall that the doctrine of the five agents was originally created to justify the violent transitions from one ruling dynasty to the next. Only later

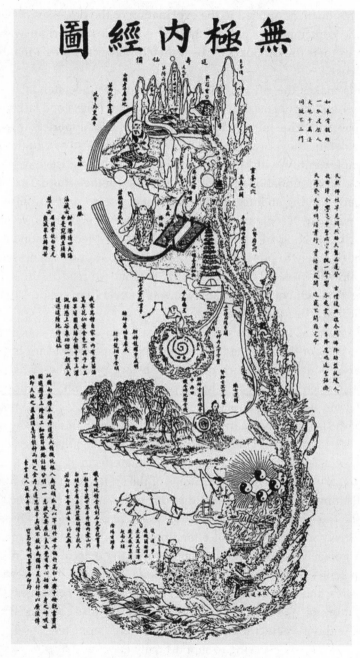

Figure 1. The human body as a landscape and village idyll in a
Daoist perspective. China, since fifteenth century.

was this doctrine applied to the explanation of the processes of nature. For the contemporary philosophers, this sociological origin was still fresh in their minds. Some of them therefore rejected it as a manmade construct.

This makes the rift that opened at that time understandable. Supporters and opponents of the idea of the complex state stood face to face. The new medicine mirrored the worldview of the supporters in almost every detail. They saw in the organism what they also saw in the state: a complex entity with different regions, all fulfilling their respective tasks on the foundation of well-defined laws, yet their mutual exchange still representing an integrated entity that appeared unified, outwardly and inwardly. Needle treatment was the intervention of choice of this medicine. Like ideal political action, the ideal needle treatment was intended solely to prevent crises, not for the therapy of sicknesses that had already broken out. At least this is what we read in the sources of the time. Of course, the requirements of everyday political life and medical practice were different.

What about medication? Here, we find two different conceptions. In the texts of the new medicine, hints about medications are certainly found—about the existence of these substances and the fact of their effects, which were apparently not overlooked after all. But such hints are few in number, and very general in nature. They change nothing about the fact that the pharmaceutics found no entry into the new medicine. The central element of integration was missing: the integration in the new science (i.e., the explanation of the effects of pharmaceutical substances) founded on the teachings of the systematic correspondence of all things. The general hints that did exist are also revealing. They ascribe the power of a ruler to substances that can heal a sickness that has already broken out. Medication kills its opponents in the organism. Such power was held only by the ruler of the empire. He confirmed death sentences each autumn. In the same manner as the ruler needs ministers and assistants, right down to the lowliest messenger boy, to stay informed and to implement his policies, one also considered medicines without distinct toxic effects to be mere "ministers," "servants," and "messengers," serving to support truly effective drugs.

21 | Pharmaceutics without Medicine

Opponents of the state idea viewed this much differently. For them, the drugs formed a central mode of therapy. The opponents also published their own political manifestos. They too attributed different levels of meaning to various drugs, and they also designated individual substances "ruler," "minister," "servant," and "messenger" to clarify their roles. But in contrast to the supporters of the new medicine, the opponents praised as "rulers" substances that were in the position to free the body from its mortal constraints and to extend the lifespan of the organism. This was their ideal: to find one's place, in societal and personal existence, in harmony with nature. To provide oneself with substances from nature, irrespective of manmade laws, and thus live a peaceful and healthy life.

Undeniably, there were still crimes in the state, just as the organism, despite good prevention, is occasionally afflicted with illness. The opponents of the state idea and of the new medicine classified those drugs used for the therapy of illness at the lowest "rank," intentionally or unintentionally using the term that also denoted the ranks of the bureaucracy. The lowest rank was comparable to the bailiffs who carried out executions of criminals. Among these delinquents were, as always, the demons and microorganisms. Both had their place in the natural environment of man. One might encounter either one just as one might encounter a snake, bear, or bird of prey. In the worldview of the healers who continued to use medical drugs, there was no reason to exclude the demons and microorganisms.

There was also no reason to now force those substances, whose effects one knew so well, into the straitjacket of the rules of systematic correspondences. Nor was there a reason to acknowledge the effects of needle treatment. Needle treatment served primarily to maintain the complex exchange system in the body. The flow between regions, the regulation of every region's contribution to the entire organism: this was the goal of the needle treatment. It comes as no surprise that those who rejected a complex state founded on such structures saw no need to adopt acupuncture as a suitable therapy form for the human organism.

Thus, the unfathomable occurred. Within one and the same Chinese culture, two therapeutic traditions originated with almost no common ground. Yet there was one exception: in 200 AD, an author named Zhang Ji tried to bridge the two traditions. To drugs, he assigned certain pathways in the body, through which they reached their sites of effectiveness. He was the first to attempt what we had taken for granted: he applied the discoveries of the new sciences to the effects of the medical substances in the body. Yet he remains an exception. No one paid attention to him. For almost a thousand years, his example found no imitators to contribute to bridging the rift. That would not happen until the eleventh century—we will return to this later.

Let us again pause to reflect for a moment. What was the foundation for the new medicine on the one hand, and for the continuation of drug therapeutics on the other? The focus of attention of both traditions was humankind. Our health was to be maintained, and, if necessary, our illnesses were to be treated. The nature of the healthy or the sick person provided no reason to choose one direction over the other. The capacity to think about the nature of things and to draw conclusions for action existed to the same extent in the followers of each respective tradition. Only the differing sociopolitical views of the holders of the two traditions were responsible for the division of Chinese therapeutics into medical and pharmaceutical traditions. These sociopolitical views conditioned respectively different worldviews, from which different views then followed about how the health and illness of the human organism should be interpreted and treated.

22 | Puzzling Parallels

Here we shall interrupt our discussion of the creation of a new medicine in Chinese antiquity. Though we have presented only part of the possible evidence, it should suffice to show how that medicine came into being. The expressive power of nature and of the human body is totally insufficient to even hint at just one of the fundamental ideas that found entrance into medicine. The expressive power of nature and of the human organism is also totally inadequate to justify the division into traditions of medicine and pharmaceutical therapeutics. Of course, both traditions were based on certain realities of morphology, physiology, and pathologic types. Yet the way these were seen, and that they were seen at all, and the way they were interpreted and used as a call to action for the prevention and therapy of illness, was laid down for scientists and physicians by social reality, not by nature.

Let us again turn to Greek antiquity. Here again, it would be very helpful to accept the thesis of the counterfeit three centuries of the Early Middle Ages. After all, it is quite strange that something totally identical to what happened in Greece happened in China three centuries later. One may assume that both events occurred independently of one another. That may well be. Or, considering the transportation situation of the time, it may have taken just that long for the innovation from the West (i.e., the Greek-influenced Eastern Mediterranean) to finally find its way to the East (i.e., China). But that can hardly be imagined. How could it have happened?

Did the impulse, on its journey to the East, stop every few hundred kilometers for a break of several decades? Were the tribes that camped along the way converted, one by one, until China was finally reached? No—back then three hundred years were just as long as they are today. There is no indication that the knowledge paused at some stopover for decades or centuries. If the transmission of certain fundamental thoughts from West to East actually occurred, then perhaps it was over the course of a few years or decades.

But if we accept this, then we have a big problem. Why would anyone, three centuries after the start of the development in Greece, travel to China to lay the foundation for a medicine that had already developed much further in Europe? Did the development in China start independently from Greece? Or may we accept the idea of the three "made-up" centuries and draw the reverse conclusion: that the development possibly started in China and radiated out to Ionia from there? A dubious assumption, since those three centuries of the Early Middle Ages cannot simply be erased from history.

Thus, a third possibility remains: the assumption that both China and the Eastern Mediterranean received external impulses that originated somewhere between the two areas and flourished, first in Greece and then later in China.

So far, we can offer neither a solution nor a meaningful assumption about how the duality of developments in East and West came about. Throughout the course of the further development of medicine in China and in the West, we repeatedly encounter quite astonishing parallels in the fundamental changes and in the awakening to new ideas.

The era of the creation of medicine in ancient Greece, which can be dated much less satisfactorily and with far fewer verifiable written sources than for that of ancient China, nevertheless allows a differentiation that has already been useful to us for our observations in China. In Greek antiquity, therapeutics were initially quite varied, supplemented by the more narrowly-defined medicine. As in China, there was no replacement of the premedical by medical therapeutics. As in China, since the creation of a medicine in ancient times, both traditions of therapeutics have existed alongside one another in Europe. That may have been very helpful for most "users" of both of these traditions. Ultimately, neither of the two traditions can claim to be perfect. Not today and even less so almost two and a half millennia ago. Both traditions, medical and nonmedical therapeutics, have had their successes. Both, however, also have their unknown territories where any approach fails.

A short examination of premedical therapeutics in Greek antiquity leads us to the work of Homer and to a few other later sources. The only theory we can recognize is the religious worldview that attributed to the gods the power to make people ill. The ancient Greeks had created the gods in their own image—only they were much more powerful. A lone person could perhaps harm and kill someone else or a small crowd of people. But Apollo could cause plague epidemics and wipe out entire populations with his arrows. In such cases, it did not occur to the ancient Greeks at all to treat patients. The aim was to soothe the rage of whomever was responsible for the plague, for with that would come healing—in this case not of the individual sick person, but of the suffering society.

It need not interest us further here that the ancient Greeks had at their disposal a variety of medicinal and mechanical interventions in the body. It is also of little interest that details of the external and internal structure of the human body are included in the works of Homer. We are concerned here with medical ideas. These, however, only began as the effort was made to free the organism, in its healthy and sick states, from the gods and to understand them solely on the basis of laws of nature. That was the beginning of medicine in Greek antiquity. This departure occurred in the fifth century BC. Before that, there was no therapeutics that comes close to our definition of medicine. Not in Greece, nor in Egypt or Mesopotamia.

The name of Hippocrates (460–ca. 380) always comes up in this context. He must have been a very impressive man—otherwise Plato would not have called him the prototype of the physician. But there is no indication that he was the creator of Greek medicine. Hippocrates was a physician of premedical therapeutics. The legend attributes no achievement to him that we could interpret as the impulse for the creation of medicine in the narrower sense. He is believed to have contributed to the teaching of therapeutics through written, documented knowledge from his time onward. This was certainly an important step. But it was not yet medicine.

The contents of the earliest writings are certainly important. Researchers now date them to the fifth century BC. The writings are concerned with the representation of observations that the attentive physician—at the time, in Greece as in China, generally an itinerant physician—could make on his travels. Here, we find the pure power of expression of the body, in health as in illness. There is no theory to come between the observer and the observed. Hippocrates cannot have espoused medicine in the sense we mean, since he was philosophically opposed to the monopolization of observation.

Two text examples substantiate the conscious attempt of some authors of the time to oppose this beginning theoreticization. We can imagine how they might have warned their students and followers: "Hold on to reality, since speculation can only lead to plausibility, not to truth!" The texts that have been handed down to us express this in a much more sophisticated and articulate manner. Thus, in the treatise "On Ancient Medicine": "I am not of the opinion that [medicine] requires a new hypothesis for invisible things about which one knows nothing . . . as there is no criteria by which the truth of the statement could be measured."[24]

The Hippocratic treatise "Instructions" defends the same approach: no theory at all! Always use visible, tangible, audible, perceptible reality for orientation: "In medicine, one must not take one's cue from theoretical considerations . . . conclusions that come from pure theory are of little use; instead use only those that are drawn from empirical observation."[25] These warnings were to no avail: they could not halt the triumphant progress of plausibility in the new medicine.

23 | The Beginning of Medicine in Greece

The origin of medicine is apparent from other ancient texts—for example, from a document with the ambitious title "The Nature of Man." This makes us sit up and take notice once again. Is the body's pure power of expression sufficient for its observer to deduce anything about the nature of man and, above all, about the nature of health and sickness? Again, as with all fundamental thoughts that found entrance into the new medicine, we must ask ourselves where these could have originated. Are the data that the body offers to the observer sufficient to arrive at such conclusions?

Let us first look at yet another text. It was dedicated to "falling sickness," or epilepsy, and discusses this under the title "The Sacred Disease," including the hitherto valid idea that, judging by the sometimes exceedingly strange course of this illness, it must be something divine, coming from the gods. This couldn't be more wrong, the author states. Falling sickness is an illness whose causes, like those of all other illnesses, lie somewhere in nature. In this case, an overabundance of phlegm in the brain causes a downflow into the body, where the pathways for blood and pneuma become blocked. This then has the known implications— the author goes into much more detail than is possible for us here.

Sounds quite right, we might agree. Not that we can fathom this phlegm obstruction theory at all. Surely we cannot. Still, the renunciation of the idea that illness is caused by the numinous powers and of the need to treat illness with magic and invocation makes sense to us. Thus we read in the literature that this is the first expression of "rational" thinking. If only it actually were.

What rational foundation could the anonymous author have had for coming up with such an idea? How could rational thinking, in the face of the terrible suffering of an epileptic, lead to such a fundamentally wrong assumption—as we know it to be today, after all—that the brain produces an excess of phlegm due to inadequate cleaning? If "rational thinking" is equated with the rejection of belief in God or in many gods, then this is a terrible insult to all those who believe in God or in many gods and who may feel quite certain in this belief, yet who are undeniably also able to think very rationally.

The author of "The Divine Illness" thought no more or less rationally than those who saw falling sickness as something divine. He had only replaced one worldview with another. At any rate, the observation of the sick individual had not produced any evidence for the new view. That was impossible. For him, only the belief was lost that the gods, whose existence he was naturally not putting into question at all, were responsible for the development of falling sickness. He lost this belief not because he had observed an epileptic, or several epileptics, or even a very large number of them. Something else must have caused his change of heart.

That is what we are interested in. Finding the impulses that, in the two millennia of the Greek and Chinese history of medicine, led to such fundamental changes of heart. The impulse was never the observation of the body. The organism's power of expression never sufficed to lead to such changes of heart. It was always the actual or aspired-to structure of human society—along with hints from nature—that provided the impulse.

24 | The End of Monarchy

Let us return to the aforementioned text on "The Nature of Man." Attributed to this text is the linking of therapeutics and the doctrine of the four humors. This would represent the origin of medicine. Two things were needed for this medicine to develop. First, the idea of laws applying to the entire universe. This condition was fulfilled. Laws comprised the foundation of society. Laws were the foundation of the macrocosm. And the *physis* itself, the individual nature of every human organism, became the embodiment of order, the epitome of regularity.[26] Next, a doctrine of laws of nature had to be applied to the human organism, to connect this organism with the regularities of its environment. This condition was met by the doctrine of the four humors.

What was this doctrine of the four humors about? Let us first take a look at the doctrine of the four elements. A man named Empedocles who lived in the fifth century is credited with the idea that no single element—water, *apeiron*, or air—can be the foundation of all life, but that the foundation is rather an equal coexistence of four elements or basic substances. Fire, water, air, and earth are all equally important for life. It is their mixture that creates life, indeed, even the entire universe.

We do not know whether Empedocles spent long years sitting at a desk with the thoughts of Thales, Anaximander, Anaximenes, and perhaps other philosophers spread before him. We also do not know whether he developed his ideas in daily discussions with other thinkers. What we do know with certainty is that he had no laboratory available where he might have conducted physiological studies on the human organism with several technical assistants performing complex measurements to identify the four basic substances in every organism and analyzing their mixture to isolate the four equal parts. So you see, what is fondly referred to as the beginning of rational science in medicine was actually sheer imagination. It was, indeed, the beginning of medicine. But this medicine can only claim to be based on reality from today's perspective. What some thinkers of the time considered truth was merely plausibility. Nothing more.

How did this plausibility come about? It would be presumptuous to seek, two and a half millennia later, an impulse for everything new. Even for later times, that would be an impossible task. Yet there is nevertheless a strange parallel between the fundamental transformations in the political environment of the thinkers who created the new medicine and the fundamental ideas of this new medicine itself.

The body disclosed no real clues that fire, water, air, and earth were its basic substances. It was sometimes hot, sometimes cold. That could count as a clue to the existence of fire in the organism. At regular intervals, the body excretes up to two liters of fluid. At irregular intervals, or under special circumstances, there are further excretions such as sweat or tears. Is this sufficient evidence for water as a basic substance for life? Possibly. After all, this water must also be supplied to the organism in appropriate amounts, or it will die of thirst. Losing too much blood also leads to death. Little needs to be said about air. We are more likely to question the idea of earth being a basic element. This is more complicated. The earth as the mother of all life, the source of all creatures—that is a longstanding view. But as a basic element? How did Empedocles find earth in the body of a person or a dog or in the cross-section of an olive tree?

We will not be able to solve this puzzle. Let us consider the statement that these four basic elements must be present to the same extent for life to exist. The four elements are on equal footing. In their mixture, they are all present in larger or smaller quantities and thereby determine the individual nature of things. But in principle, they are all always present and control existence. Thus, they stand in opposition to the older thinking of Thales, Anaximander, and Anaximenes, each of whom had recognized only one element, one basic substance, as governing life.

These metaphors have not been chosen unintentionally here. The only parallel we can discern for these changed ideas about the foundations and basic elements of life is the transformation of the social structure from monarchy to democracy. Alcmaeon of Croton (ca. 570–500) is the chief witness. As a physician and philosopher, he knew what he was talking about. He created the doctrine of isonomy. Literally, he referred to the *isonomia ton dynameon*, the equal standing of the powers. One might say he spoke of a balance of power. In referring to the physical organism, he used terms normally used for the social organism. This is familiar to us from China. The physical organism is healthy when all parts are present in a well-balanced mixture. The opposite of this is *monarchia*, "the rule of one." *Monarchia*, he pointed out so clearly, is an illness.

The origins of monistic thought possibly lie in Asia. From there, this idea may have found entrance to Ionia and then to Greece. In view of the political shift to polis democracy, it could apparently no longer preserve itself. It is difficult to explain why four was the number of choice in the Eastern Mediterranean. Speculation about an impulse from Persia is helpful, but insufficient. We can merely determine that, in the fifth century BC, the Greeks were victorious over the Persians and could contrast oriental despotism and their own monarchical past with the culture of debate and persuasion, and so the structures of the polis democracy matured. This was a fundamental change in their living environment.

Though not all political goals ripened into lasting reality, as ideals they influenced the thinking and aspirations of many. Who should then be surprised that the general shift to polis democracy and rule of law caused some thinkers to attribute the power over health and illness no longer to the gods, but instead to the lawfulness of natural processes? The author of "The Divine Illness" did not of his own accord think more rationally than his predecessors. Like the others, he was led to see things in a new way and to include a detail like epilepsy in a new worldview.

Not everyone thought this way. Indeed, a new cult even originated, the cult of Asclepius, who was believed to be a divine person able to heal those who faithfully came to him and fell asleep in his temple, like a kind autocrat relieving people from illness. The Asclepius cult was not a short-lived uprising of a fading mentality. Quite the contrary, it persisted throughout antiquity as an important part of therapeutics as a whole—and it was not only the less intelligent, the less thoughtful, or the formally less educated who hoped for help from such therapy.

Neither Greece nor China ever produced a therapeutic monoculture. People with varying experiences, worldviews, and life plans always lived alongside each other. These experiences, worldviews, and life plans corresponded to varying interpretations of the sick and healthy organism. Yet it should be emphasized that it would be plainly impossible to trace back every interpretation to the personal experiences and life circumstances of those who expressed them. Too many overlapping layers blur the picture. All we can do is attempt to answer the question whether the fundamental ideas of medicine originate from the expressive power of the body or from other impulses influencing the contemplative observer.

25 | Troublemakers and Ostracism

The doctrine of the four elements could not have originated in the expressive power of the body itself. The same holds true for the doctrine of the four humors. Supposedly, a man named Polybos introduced it toward the end of the fifth century BC, applying it consistently to the assessment of the human organism, or to be more precise, to the explanation of health and illness. Polybos, if it was actually he, did not, it should be emphasized, introduce the doctrine of the four humors into medicine! Indeed, a medicine into which he could have introduced this doctrine did not even exist yet. He—or whoever achieved this step—was the first to fulfill the basic condition for the creation of medicine. He was the first to base the interpretation of the human conditions of sickness and health purely on the laws of nature and thus on a scientific foundation. Whoever introduced the doctrine of the four humors into therapeutics was the creator of the first medicine in the history of humankind!

This step was definitely not prompted by the expressive power of the body. That much is certain. But it was complemented by the body's own expressiveness! This is how fundamental progress came about in ancient medicine and also in the medicine of the following centuries up to the present. The impulse for new thinking always came from outside the body. First came changes in the social structures in which the Greeks lived or aspired to live. Structures triggering a shift in thinking can be real or ideal—actually prevailing or fervently aspired to. The structures that led to the rethinking in ancient Greece were those of the polis democracy.

On this, the historian of medicine Georg Harig has appropriately noted: "For the first time in human history, polis democracy approached man as a political individual, brought from anonymity into the center of social events, and the pervasive concept of society as a community of equal individuals was promoted. This development created the social backdrop for the pursuits of scientific Greek medicine, with its rigorously individualizing progress." It may be a bit exaggerated to claim that all individuals in the polis community were seen as equal. Surely Harig's statement referred only to free citizens and in the end applies only to them. The ranks of these citizens, the self-image of these citizens, the political awareness of these citizens, the destiny of the polis, the fate of their social organism—this was the backdrop for the emergence of the ideas that, via the new worldview and understanding of nature, finally flowed into therapeutics and created the first new medicine.

The monistic or, to put it bluntly, "monarchistic" view of the "rulers" of a fundamental element must have naturally yielded to the new view of a larger number, in this case a quartet, of basic parts to a living organism. Whether it is four or five or six is trivial. The important thing is that the idea prevailed that several fundamental elements carried, in their mixture, a complex structure and thus made life possible for this structure. The details come from the graphic nature of the body. After the basic structures imposed themselves from the outside onto the body like a matrix, the reality of the body could deliver material to fill up the fundamental structures.

Water, fire, air, and earth were too general, too vague. What did the healer really see? He saw blood, mucus, yellow bile, and black bile. And he also saw that in some situations, blood flow was increased or the vessels were more swollen than usual. Such situations were felt to be unpleasant. They were considered to be abnormal because they injured the aesthetic of the handsome, pleasant-smelling person, and perhaps because they were a hindrance to normal daily routine. The ancient healer saw that excessive mucus or yellow or black humors flowed out of all sorts of body openings. That was all. Exactly the same principle was at work here as in the state: Only a balance of all those involved can guarantee harmony and peace in the polis. Only a balance of all the humors and elements can guarantee health in the human organism. Any excess is harmful. *Medèn agàn* was the Greek equivalent of the Chinese doctrine of the mean. It originated in the social realm and of course also found entrance into the view of the organism.

Excess has consequences. Harmful substances can arise from the wrong mixture of the basic substances. Take pus, for example. It must leave the community of "good" basic elements. It is the same with all other harmful substances that are not required by the organism because all they can do is mischief. The body discharges these harmful substances. The ostracism that takes place somewhere in the interior of the body cannot be seen. But the result is only too clear. The polis did this, too. Whoever did not fit in was discharged. He might even be killed. No less a man than Socrates had to experience this. In any case, the actual or supposed pest had to go away. The body also does this. Rejection, apostasis, is the natural method of freeing itself of harmful substances. If the body itself cannot manage this, the physician must intervene and help. Vomiting might help. Purging, sweating, bloodletting might help. And if there is just no other way, one must be brave enough to apply the knife.

We are now at a point where medicine can believe in itself. Here it can have an opinion, to defend its own ideas—about the healthy and sick conditions of the organism and of the best healing methods—in its own right. Here, medicine can claim that it is legitimated by nothing but a view on the body itself. No doubt, there will always be a few spoilsports. And not just late in the game, but right from the outset. Thus it is reported that Heraclites and Empedocles did not at all approve of continually making new judgments about the condition of the organism on the basis of new observations.

What did Empedocles need observations for, anyway? It seems that he came to his realizations purely by thinking, and that although this had little to do with reality, it has guaranteed him immortality up to the present and surely into the distant future. Of course, he could not totally do without the expressive power of the body. Fire, water, air, and earth had to be in balance. Too much fire chases the water out. He must have experienced this often himself, sweating in the heat. Cooling causes many movements to slacken and grow weary. Cold ultimately means the end of all movement: death.

26 | I See Something You Don't See

Such attempts at explanation were an easy game for Empedocles. But he also tackled more difficult problems. What is the interplay of blood and breath? It was obvious that a kind of movement must occur in the body. Some ancient Chinese observers had suggested circulation both of qi, the most finely dispersed, breathlike material, and blood. This was not the circulation recognized by the Englishman William Harvey (1578–1657) over one and a half millennia later. But nevertheless, blood and qi flowed through a complex system of vessels, here and there, to and fro, and early Chinese authors described two closed circulations in the body: one each on the left and right sides, in which the flow proceeded as in a ring, without beginning or end.

This sounds modern, but it is not. At first, it was simply the application of the circulation of the national economy to the idea of the necessity of supplying the body regions. As so often in the history of medicine, speculation then immediately broke away from the concrete example. It gained a momentum of its own and created its own models, with few recognizable details of the original impulse. However, the important thing in comparing Greek and Chinese dealings with blood and qi (or breath) is that the new, breakthrough idea of circulation that Chinese thinkers had in antiquity did not come about in Greek antiquity.

Let us again recall the hypothesis that has been the basis of our discussions so far. People have long been basically the same in appearance. Physical differences such as nose shape or skin color are irrelevant here. In addition, the observers are basically the same everywhere. An ancient Greek philosopher was exactly as intelligent and similarly worldly as his Chinese colleague. Why then should one of them see something in the human organism that the other could not see? This question poses itself not only in comparison of the cultures of ancient Greece and ancient China, so distant from one another. It also poses itself within one and the same culture—close together in time and place—and also in later eras. It poses itself, for example, in light of the fact that in the second half of the nineteenth century, the accomplished university professor Rudolf Virchow (1821–1902) could not at all see what the equally accomplished district physician Robert Koch (1843–1910) saw, that is, that tuberculosis was caused by a very specific pathogen. The question becomes even more explosive if we reformulate it with a view to the debate on the circulation of blood and qi: Why should someone see something in the human organism that does not exist in reality, and why would someone else not see the same thing? This is the question that sets us on the right track.

Why did the ancient Greeks see no circulation? They saw vessels and described them in detail. After all, the fluids in the body, particularly the four humors, had to reach all the regions. One would surely have seen some real vessels. It cannot be said on what occasions. But most of what the ancient Greeks wrote about this was meticulously thought out. It was in keeping not with the limited power of expression of the body, but with the logic of the humors doctrine. It was plausibility, not reality. In China as well, the focus was on vessels long before an ancient version of the idea of circulation had been formulated there. But to assume that the vessels were associated with such a circulation was by no means a matter of course. It had to be thought up. And for that, there had to be an impulse.

Was there no impulse at all for this reality that the ancient Greeks might have stumbled across in their social or natural environment? Well, more than half a millennium later, in the second century AD, the celebrated Galen of Pergamon (ca. 129–199), active mostly in Rome, thought up what he called the small circulation. But we are getting ahead of ourselves. Empedocles was probably the first to attempt an explanation. He envisioned a purely mechanical movement of blood and air in the body. He oriented himself only toward the mechanics of the pipette. No other inspiration came to him. This is noteworthy.

In China, we recognized the idea of the circulation in the body as a projection of the circulation in the unified, multicentric state. The political terminology preferred by early medical authors in China makes the source of the impulses quite clear. Empedocles had no such model before his eyes. He saw only what was most obvious. That was the pipette. His unambitious model more or less said the following: There are vessels in the body. Blood moves in them. When it flows downward, the blood leaves an emptiness in the vessels. Into this emptiness, air immediately flows, inhaled through the human mouth and nose. When blood again ascends and refills the spaces filled with air, the air must escape. This is evident when one exhales.

Thus the Chinese, through their choice of terminology, identified the national economy of the unified kingdom as the impulse. Thus Empedocles himself named the pipette as his model image. That is the correct term. From the model image of the pipette, he created what he considered a realistic image of the processes in the body. Perhaps he was not aware that he had also included the eternal process of ebb and flow among his model images. Perhaps he had once, without remembering it, observed the seaside spectacle that continues to fascinate today's tourists. On the rocky coast, crashing waves cause foam and water to spray out of narrow chasms and abysses, an impressive picture of the unrelenting exchange of water and air in these cavities.

Can we thus assume that the Chinese saw something in the body that the Greeks did not, because the Chinese had a model image that the Greeks simply lacked? Sometimes the parallels between what one finds in the philosophical writings of the two cultures are so plainly disclosed that one hardly dares to compare them. But let us attempt it very carefully here. In the Daoist classic the *Dao De Jing* (attributed to Laozi—also spelled Laotse or Lao-tzu among other variations) is a lovely summary of thoughts on how ideal social life should be structured. This ideal was certainly not the complex, multicentric state characterized by the exchange of goods among people, its details regulated by a literate bureaucracy. Chapter 80 of the *Dao De Jing* contains an alternative concept:

> Let there be a small land with few inhabitants, people who would not use new inventions even if they reduced the work by ten or a hundred times, people twice as likely to die than emigrate. Boats and wagons might exist, but no one would ride in them; weapons might exist, but no one would learn to use them. People would know of no other writing than knots in ropes, be content with their food and happy with their clothes and their shelter and take delight in their simple customs. The next community might be close enough to hear their rooster crowing and their dogs barking, but people would grow old and die never having gone there.[27]

No state worthy of the name can be founded on such ideas. It is thus not surprising that other social philosophies won the race for the ruler's favor in the newly unified Chinese kingdom. But what is the link to Greece? It can be found in two things. First, those Chinese observers of the human body who espoused the Daoist ideas of an ideal societal structure did not see the circulation that the physicians postulated, whose ideas were marked by Confucian and/or Legalistic thought. These people may have lived with and alongside each other, in one and the same society, but they played the game of "I see something you don't see!"

No two parties could play this game in Greece. At the time, there was no model image that some saw while others did not. In Greek antiquity, as Empedocles and others formulated their ideas and profound doctrines there was no explicit model image of a great social circulation as there was in China following the unification of the kingdom. Unambiguity is one precondition, revolutionary newness another, for the model image to change into the new view of the organism, whether the model image is real or ideal.

To explain this smooth parallel, let us quote Kitto, the scholar of antiquity, one last time: "The modern reader who concerns himself with political philosophers as utterly foreign to him as Plato or Aristotle is impressed with how much they insist that the polis must be economically self-sufficient. To them, self-sufficiency is really the first precondition for the existence of the polis. If everything went according to them, trade could be done away with completely."[28] Brothers in spirit—at least in this respect—with the author of the *Dao De Jing*.

Kitto asks the question that almost forces itself on us in comparison with China: "But why did such cities not form larger units?" And he answers it right away: "Initially, there was an economic reason. The geographic barriers with which Greece is so richly endowed impeded the transport of goods by any other than the sea route, which was still insecure. In addition, the multiformity of the land made it possible to provide for one's self fairly well in quite small areas, particularly for a people making such low material demands of life as the Greeks. Both fostered the same development. The individual parts of the land were neither economically dependent on one another, nor did they attract each other."[29] Ah, if only we had more exact information on which western land it was that, according to the legend, Laozi rode to from China on his water buffalo at the end of his life! In the polis of Greece, with its undemanding, frugal inhabitants, he might have felt right at home.

Now we can see things more clearly. Those Chinese who lived in the thought world of the national economic structures of the complex empire played the game of "I see something you don't see" not only with those that lived within their own culture (i.e., those who were blind to circulation in the body), but also with the Greeks, who lived three hundred years earlier and possessed no model image at all from which they might have derived a view of the circulation in the body. The Daoist thinkers of China neither wanted nor were able to see the model image—impressive as it nevertheless was—and thus had no impulse for the idea of circulation.

At no time did the Greek observers have a model image—neither. in the real existing societal structure nor as an ideal, aspired-to vision. Thus they had no chance at all to escape from Empedocles' rudimentary pipette model. Eventually, in the seventeenth century, William Harvey first recognized and described the circulation of blood in the dimensions still recognized today. The irony of the story is that he also needed a model image as he searched for and found what we consider reality. His model image was Aristotle's idea of rotation in nature. Why Aristotle himself never came up with the idea of a circulation of blood, air, or pneuma in the body is one of the puzzles whose solution history will perhaps forever deny us.

One might object that Harvey could only come up with his description of circulation after the discovery of lung circulation and on the foundation of knowledge of the vein valves and many other previous achievements. That is true if we emphasize that Harvey first created the physiologically and morphologically basically correct interpretation of the movement of blood. It is, however, not true that all this previous knowledge was needed to develop the thesis of a great circulation of blood flowing through the entire body. Ancient China gives us the proof for that. Then why not also Aristotle, who was really so close?

An explanation might go something like this: the Chinese who saw circulation in the body had the circulation of goods and people in their complex state as a model. Harvey, who also saw circulation in the body, had a great amount of actual knowledge at his disposal. Thus he was able, through impulses from his readings of Aristotle and other philosophers, to link up all of this, to initially suspect the right solution and then to scientifically prove it. But Aristotle and other early Western thinkers had neither the one nor the other. They had no model image in the social structures in which they lived or that they aspired to, and they had no appropriate actual knowledge that merely needed to be summarized brilliantly. What did they have? Just the pipette.

27 | Powers of Self-healing: Self-evident?

The game of "I see something you don't see" would be played again, but in the reverse direction, for there were also phenomena seen by the Greeks but not by the Chinese. To be more precise, both the Chinese and the Greeks saw something, but only the Greeks discerned what they saw and looked beyond it for something more, which is what the Chinese, for their part, did not see. This sounds more complicated than it actually is, since it was known to both the Chinese and the Greeks that a certain proportion of human illness sometimes takes a turn for the better without any human therapeutic influence. Today we speak, for example, of the self-healing of a horrible sickness or of a spontaneous remission. In Greek antiquity, a healing power of its own was attributed to the *physis*, or human nature.

And with that, we are at the center of our topic of interest. The Greeks saw that illnesses can heal by themselves. And not only a small wound that closes itself seemingly on its own. Even the most terrible cancers sometimes unexpectedly take a turn for the better, without any recognizable external cause. In Greece and beyond, in contrast to China, this observation provoked an endless chain of theories on the reasons behind such self-healings. The ancient dictum *nouson physieis ietroi* says that every organism possesses its own authority, its *physis*, which is the true physician for the illnesses of this body. The human physician, so it is argued by the defenders of this generally accepted thesis, is really only required when the "natural" physician residing in the body cannot cope.

The so-called self-healing powers of the body are worthy of our attention. They represent nothing other than the certainty that the body has a self-interest and—this is especially important—its own capacity to pull itself out of crisis and restore a condition of harmony. You might wonder what is so special about this, seeing as there is simply no other explanation at all. With such a comment, you would merely reveal yourself as being tied up in Western traditions of thought. For that is the fascinating thing about the wealth of information on the history of medicine in Europe and in China: we can make comparisons. Something one or the other side accepts as given may be questioned by the other. This is the case with the idea of self-healing powers—they are, in fact, not at all as obvious as it might appear to those of us who were raised in the Western tradition. Their existence has, at any rate, never been proven.

We can only suspect—as we have done since antiquity—that the organism possesses a built-in teleology of harmony, that is to say, that it single-mindedly strives for its own well-being. As long as the problem or illness is not too severe, the organism will find a way out of this situation and restore its health. Yet it is strange that this was noticed only by the Europeans and not by the Chinese. Granted, there are also other possible solutions to the enigma of self-healing. For example, the idea that everyone has a guardian angel or ancestors watching over him and possibly keeping him alive. Neither one (the idea of self-healing powers) nor the other (the idea of guardian angels or ancestors) can be proven or disproven. The only difference is that for most observers since the beginning of scientific medicine two millennia ago, plausibility lies on the side of the self-healing powers. Other Europeans, much less influential in the field of medicine, are convinced of the existence of guardian angels or other numinous powers bringing salvation to those in a hopeless situation.

28 | Confucians' Fear of Chaos

Thus we again return to the questions that will occupy us further: Where did the impulse for the observation of the self-healing powers originate? What model image elicited the idea that the organism possesses a self-interest and an ability to lead itself out of crisis? Here again, mere observation of the body was not nearly enough. Following the observation of the body, Greek and Chinese medics could say only that some illnesses seem to get better on their own. This is all the body says. Everything else is an idea that the observer creates, and for this idea he needs a model image. Was there such a model image in the Greek environment of the polis democracy? Indeed, there was. And it is not difficult to find.

The body as an organism has self-interest and tries to heal its own wounds and overcome difficult crises on its own: this idea is based on the model image of the self-regulating, autonomous polis. The polis had transformed itself from the monarchy and the rule of the noble families into a democratic structure that was optimal for the situation of the time, a democracy in which the citizens were the sovereigns of their own fates through their meetings. Ideally, they would need no overriding ruler. Rational discussions were their ideal solution to crises. Of course, crises could grow out of hand to the extent that one might be grateful to a "tyrant" like Peisistratus for temporarily directing the course of events single-handedly.

The polis was a social organism. It was entirely unavoidable that its structures lent the plausibility needed for the explanatory model of the self-healing powers to find general acceptance. Over the course of two millennia, Western physicians have often presented cases of incredible transformations from terminal illness to recovery without any recognizable intervention. The interest has been sustained in Western medicine, interpreting this phenomenon of self-healing in the sick organism. We know that the organism occasionally cures itself. We just do not know how.

And in China? What model image could have there been for inspiring a similar idea? The fact that sicknesses—many of them, in fact—heal on their own is also described repeatedly in the ancient Chinese literature. For the most part, we find the laconic statement "do not treat, heals on its own." In contrast to the ancient Greek literature, the ancient Chinese literature does not contain descriptions of the course of a normally fatal illness taking an unanticipated and unexpected turn for the better. Why some sicknesses heal on their own has never been an issue in the history of Chinese medicine, again in clear contrast with Europe.

Thus, no one came up with an idea similar to that of Greek antiquity.

Quite simply, the model image was missing. Never in its history, from antiquity to the twentieth century, did Chinese society have democratic structures. These would not be imported from the West and imposed on an unprepared culture until the twentieth century. The republic that attempted democracy fled to the island of Taiwan after World War II. The mainland has since been continuing the two-thousand-year-old tradition of authoritarian rule. Where could there ever have been a model image for the idea of the organism as a self-governing, self-healing structure? China has never been ruled democratically. China has never known trust in the self-regulating powers of the pan-societal organism. It has never had a ruling structure in which citizens discuss their conflicting interests and even in crisis seek an amicable solution.

Chinese traditional medicine faithfully mirrors the authoritarian structures of antiquity. Neither Confucian-Legalistic social philosophy nor the opposing social teachings of Daoism were in any way democratic. Both emphasized the role of the ruler or autocrat as being responsible for the fate of the masses. The differences were in the details. For the Legalists, the ruler stood above the law. Other philosophers saw the ruler as subject to the law. But the only known form of society had a single ruler at the top. The Confucians in particular were, as Leipzig Sinologist Ralf Moritz so precisely expressed it, practically possessed by a "fear of chaos." That is to say that chaos (the word for political unrest) was to be prevented at all costs.

The wise men of antiquity, writes the philosopher Xunzi, did not wait to intervene to restore order once chaos or unrest had already broken out. They already intervened to promote order when there was no chaos at all, no foreseeable unrest. A bit further into the first great text of the new Chinese medicine, we again read the same wording—extended only by the statement that the wise men of antiquity also brought illnesses back to order not once they had already broken out, but by treating the illness before it had come into existence. In other words, in a case of unrest and crisis, society can never be trusted to find the path to peace and harmony on its own. In a case of sickness, the human organism can never be trusted to find the path to health on its own.

One might object that this statement opposes the observation that illnesses occasionally do not require therapy because they heal on their own! This indeed posed a difficult question for the ancient observers in China, who were strongly influenced by their authoritarian ruling structures. Yet they solved it easily. First of all, they simply did not observe any unexpected spontaneous remissions. Consequently, they did not describe such courses of illness. The Greek physician, in contrast, was very familiar with such situations. He even waited for the organism of his patient to help itself. He observed his sick patient to see whether things would take a turn for the better on their own. Particularly with a more serious illness, one could never be sure. Only in the most urgent emergency was outside help necessary.

In ancient Chinese literature, the only self-healings described are those that were expected from the outset. There are no unexpected self-healings. The recognized self-healings were indeed seen, but they caused no ongoing debate on reasons. Overall, there is only a single line of reasoning from antiquity—and it is typically Chinese. That is, it completely corresponds with the model image a contemporary observer had in mind when he imagined what was happening in the organism.

The solution was simple: illnesses stem from conflicts among the various parties in the organism. The interests of these parties are sufficiently well-known. There were some parties, convincingly explained in the context of the doctrine of the five agents, who would kill each other if they had the chance. Of course, there were also those who created each other, like a mother and her son. The physician diagnosing an illness must, like a wise ruler, determine the nature of the conflict playing itself out deep inside the organism. If these are two parties that behave like a mother and son, he can relax. Nothing is going to happen. As a rule— and Confucian moralists assumed that these rules would be followed—a mother and her son do not hurt each other. The occasional argument is inevitable. It happens all the time, even in the best of families. But to kill each other? No, not that. So why intervene? The problem will resolve itself.

But then it is also possible that two parties come into conflict and really want to kill each other. In such cases, early intervention is necessary. Such a conflict cannot be resolved once it has broken out and catastrophe is then unavoidable. The clever physician, like the wise ruler, must intervene in such cases and exercise his authority to promote order. That is the only solution. In China there is no trust in the self-regulating potential of the organism—neither the societal nor the bodily organism. Where no model image was to be found in the actual or aspired-to social structure, no corresponding image of the structures in the human organism could develop. The self-healing powers were not an issue. I see something you don't see—the Greeks did not see circulation; the Chinese saw no self-healing.

29 | Medicine: Expression of the General State of Mind

We are now generally acquainted with the fundamental ideas of the newly created medicine in Chinese and Greek antiquity. We have seen that the human body itself offers no sufficient image of its organic functions and malfunctions to elicit the statements that the new medicine created, in both cultural domains. We have also seen that there were obviously model images to be found not in the body, but in the structure of the prevailing social conditions—actual or idealized. These model images gave the impulses that guaranteed the plausibility of the theories of the normal and the abnormal, that is, of the healthy and the sick processes in the body. The expressive power of the body—with its morphological details, its temperature and color changes, its smells and excretions—is extremely limited. It is not the body's power of expression that leads to the creation of medical doctrine. Rather, doctrines stimulated by the model images outside the body serve to explain the information that the body itself can make available.

In conclusion, let us take another comparative look at Chinese and Greek medicine. Chinese medicine was created in an environment that recognized the exchange between various regional centers as the foundation of a new state organism, the unified empire. Also of great importance for Confucian society was the regulated order of relationships between well-defined social poles: ruler and subjects, father and son, older brother and younger brother, husband and wife, and friend and friend. For two millennia, these ideas of regulated relationships of various individual parts remained the foundation of the Confucian-influenced society. For two millennia, the idea of the relationships of various functional centers in the human organism was the most important feature of Chinese medicine. The morphological structure of the individual parts involved in the exchange was of less interest than the guarantors of well-being—the ordered relationships and the exchange among the involved functional centers.

We refer to the teachings about these relationships in ancient Chinese medicine as the doctrine of systematic correspondences. Within a short period of time, the yin-yang and five agents doctrines were further elaborated by many authors to such an extent that their representation here would require many pages. So far, there are no complete portrayals of these theories in any Western language—neither in their early dimensions nor in their later, increasingly comprehensive applications.

The Greek medical theorists also considered the doctrine of correspondences, but it was of less importance. The doctrines of the four elements, the four humors and a few other corresponding groups of four were kept very short. Historians of medicine can present them exhaustively in one page or in just a few pages. In China, one has the impression that the yin-yang and five agents doctrines of the systematic relationships of all phenomena had the support and approval of part of the elite. These doctrines obviously resounded with the basic sentiments of these people and therefore found—probably unintentionally and unnoticed—their reflection in the medicine that this elite created for itself. In Greece, the doctrine of the four correspondences seems more like a compulsory exercise. Perhaps it was triggered by an external impulse. It was in no way followed as consistently as in China.

Greek medicine was created in an environment that recognized the autarchy of small political units as the foundation of a new state organism, the polis democracy. The exchange between various centers was of marginal importance. The significant thing was the individual center. Perhaps the significance of relationships among individuals had less prominence in Greek antiquity compared to the emphasis on such relationships in China. There is no doubt that in ancient Greece there were also considerations of the fundamental relationships among people. Aristotle identified such basic relationships as the sexual relationship between man and woman, the work relationship between master and slave, and the relationship of father (parents) and children in need of help. But these social relationships are much more specific and narrowly defined than those Confucianism considered to be fundamental for morality.

Another point to keep in mind is that Confucianism based its teachings of the five fundamental relationships on a moral upbringing that affected every educated person. Aristotle's teaching of the three basic relationships did not have such broad repercussions. Additionally, if we would like to trace the main features of ancient medicine to nonmedical impulses, we will not necessarily find this in the works of individual philosophers. Certain aspects may correspond with individual philosophical works. Overall, however, medicine mirrors a more comprehensive state of mind that was either shared by the entire elite of the time or, as we have seen in China, influenced at least part of the elite.

Thus, if we would like to understand the origin of the importance of the individual morphological body part in Greek medicine, we will not find the answer in Aristotle, Epicurus, or another representative of one of the great competing schools of thought. We must search for those ideological aspects that united the creators of the medicine that shaped the particular orientation of Greek medicine. The philosophical aspects that led the focus of Greek medicine, in contrast to Chinese medicine, to emphasize the physical substrate may have to do with the fact that in Greek antiquity, the individual part seemed more important than any relationships between individual parts.

It is important to remember that Chinese medicine tended to emphasize the interplay of functions while Western medicine was, into the twentieth century, primarily interested in the illumination of morphological details. This can be traced back to the initial influence on the two thought systems. In both China and Greece, antiquity had laid the foundation for the kind of medicine that would prevail for the following two millennia. Not until the twentieth century were there fundamental changes in both traditions—even if, overall, these can hardly be seen as innovations.

New to Western medicine was the insight into the complete networking of all body parts and functions through biochemical and biophysical pathways. Not until the twentieth century did Western medicine create a kind of systematic correspondence comprising the entire body. Of course, the X—the intangible, invisible spirit—was still missing. For Chinese medicine, the adoption of Western medicine was the decisive innovation of the twentieth century. Along with this adoption came the need to redefine Chinese medicine and adapt to Western science in theory and practice. Thus, after two millennia of mostly separate histories, a new phase began for both medical traditions, one that fundamentally changed both healing systems. But more on that later.

30 | Dynamic Ideas and Faded Model Images

The new medicines in both Greece and China took their model images from their creators' living environments. The new medicine had an idea of the body, but the model image for it was not the body itself—at least not for the fundamental assumption that if certain things happen inside the body, a person will be healthy or get sick. The body, or, to be more precise, the reality of the body, certainly played a role in this. Blood, mucus, urine, and stool could be seen. Abnormal temperatures of people who were sick, had fevers, or were cold after death could be felt. Colors and smells changed. Swelling, bumps, and ulcers appeared before the eyes of the observers. Pain could create havoc anywhere in the body. So, it was certainly not as if the body had nothing to communicate. On the contrary, it communicated much and, by all its conspicuous signs, gave a first impulse for interpretation. But the body can only provide descriptions of condition. The body can only give clues: A sore throat. A swollen belly. Hair falling out. An ulcer flaring up. The body says nothing about the organism. It is the task of X to ultimately clarify what the body is and how the organism functions in this body.

We have seen the results of this thinking, the creation of the first medicine. But what happened next? Time did not simply stand still. The polis democracies soon ceased to exist. By the fourth century, their era had passed. Still, they had provided the model image for the idea of the organism in the new medicine. What effects did losing the model image have on the further existence of the new medicine? How can a medicine survive once the model image has been lost?

Here, we have reached a decisive point. Repeatedly throughout the history of medicine, model images were lost. However, this is not to say that the idea of the organism that had emerged from this model image likewise disappeared. The idea took on a life of its own. It became fixed, recorded in writing, taught to students—with a tenacity that long outlasted the model image itself.

Once a theory is put down in writing, it is released from the original model and gains a dynamic of its own. People logically discuss the arguments of the doctrine. The original impulse for creating this doctrine retreats into the background and becomes unimportant. The doctrine carries itself. Writings are passed down from generation to generation. Students have to learn the doctrines and later teach them to their own students. But the idea system is nevertheless an open one. Again and again, a few thoughtful individual practitioners appear on the scene who can also observe. They find contradictions between what they have learned and what they have experienced.

They correct the theory—sometimes only in small ways, and sometimes with a breakthrough. Then, things become difficult. Does the breakthrough rest only on one's own world view? In that case, the new idea of the organism and its creator will soon fade and be forgotten. The works of such authors are lined up alongside each other like gravestones in the cemetery of medical history. There are countless such gravestones. Exhuming these would at most be of interest to archeologists of knowledge. However, if the breakthrough is founded on a worldview, on life experience, on structures of social existence or fervently aspired-to forms of existence shared by many or even everyone in a society, then the new idea is sure to have plausibility, and it will outlive its creator.

This is not to say that it will convince everyone else. Someone who was intensively trained in his childhood and youth to adhere to a system of ideas is unlikely to separate himself from it later on. Society's transition from an old to new worldview is smoother. Sudden departures from the old doctrine are exceedingly rare. Old and new reside alongside one another, each eyeing the other critically. The great variety of therapeutic systems has its origin not only in the fact that various groups with different worldviews live together in the same society, but it has also developed through the tenacity of idea systems that, once introduced, separated from their model image and survived on their own.

31 | The Hour of the Dissectors

In 323 BC, Alexander the Great died. His great empire broke apart into four kingdoms. Of them, only Alexandria is of relevance to us. It was to Alexandria that the center of Greek learning and hunger for knowledge shifted. Here, the hypothesis that our discussion is based on must pass its first test. The polis democracy was long since history. Alexander's father, King Philip of Macedonia, knew that it had already outlived itself when he took advantage of the discord in Athens for his conquests. Now, in the new center of a completely different political structure, nothing fit together anymore. But there were those who continued with the old way, who did not notice that they were clinging to dead branches whose roots had dried up. No new life could flow into the branches. But it did not matter. They had books. A few people thought and wrote on the established foundation. Their patients were also quite satisfied with this.

And yet, the change in the environment immediately made itself obvious. For example, there was a man named Herophilus of Chalcedon (ca. 335 BC), to whom later ancient authors attributed a very active interest in anatomical studies. He came close to reality and forged further ahead than anyone before him. He conducted postmortem examinations, looking at the brain, eyes, digestive organs, and vessels. He observed the female and male sexual organs with interest—internally and externally. What did he see? He saw the old humoral teachings corroborated. The body only revealed its external appearance, even if it was on the inside. There were no new impulses. What new thing could Herophilus have discovered besides some astonishing morphological details?

There was yet another contemporary: Erasistratus of Julis on Chios (ca. 300–240 BC). It was said of him and other corpse dissectors that they even cut open living bodies. Erasistratus had a special interest in the nerves and vessels. He searched for the transport paths for pneuma throughout the organism. He compared living bodies and corpses. This brought him quite close to reality. How else could he have claimed that the heart is the origin of all movement of fluids and pneuma?

Several decades ago, Ludwig Edelstein came up with an explanation of this stormy development in Alexandria. His conclusions are still worth reading today. Two things came together. First, the close connection between the human being and the universe broke apart. We have seen this before. Greek ideas of the linking of all things, of the systematic correlation of all phenomena, were really quite meager, especially compared with what the Chinese created a little later. It was halfhearted in the Eastern Mediterranean region, and it did not last long. As Alexander's kingdom broke apart, the idea of the unity of the human being and the cosmos, weak to begin with, soon disappeared. Those who hitherto had not wanted to look at the human body on the inside, assuming they would see the same thing as in animals, would now learn better. The second thing was that the focus of attention now shifted to the human body.

Alexandria rapidly developed into a glittering catwalk of vanities. It became a true center of world trade, where much money, wealth, and power assembled. The image cultivation and self-promotion of the ruler and his surroundings was new to the Greeks. Even in the firmament, the hierarchy changed: for the first time—even if only temporarily—the sun moved into the center of the worldview. This was inevitable. Alone, it would not have been enough for the human body to become the object of curiosity and of the thirst for knowledge. A corresponding philosophy was necessary for this. The great Greek thinker Aristotle (384–322) was in keeping with the times. He exhorted everyone to go directly to the object! To look at it oneself. It was important to not always only brood about reality from a distance, but rather to study it at close range. But to confront the human body directly? Even to cut it open? Aristotle delivered the right argument at the right time: There is absolutely nothing human about the corpse! The soul is what is truly human. It is safe to separate body and soul. So go on, what are you waiting for?

Do we remember the life formula? Aristotle's idea was already quite bold: Life = body + X. Aristotle moved that which is human into the X. He attributed nothing human to the body devoid of X. He threw it to the dissectors. Herophilus, Erasistratus, and others did not have to be told twice. They began cutting open even living felons. Perhaps it could be seen how the X, and with it humanness, escapes from the body?

This looking around in the body did not suit everyone. To some thoughtful observers of nature, anatomy was too closely linked with the old theories. They called for a radical departure. Forget all this interpretation! Illness is real. Medicines that can end illness are likewise real. Nothing more is needed. Everything else is speculation. The plausibility of theory is not needed. The empiricists, as these skeptics were called, built their knowledge on only two pillars of experience: observation of the effects of medicine and observation of the course of illness. They considered it illegitimate to go beyond that. Antiquity thanks them for the development of pharmacy.

Do we recall? It is indeed astonishing. In ancient China, about three centuries later, some intellectuals broke free from the theory of the new medicine. It was the same group within the elite that had been engaged in the empirical, pragmatic application and further development of pharmacy. Likewise, in Alexandria, some intellectuals rejected theory. Unfortunately, we know nothing about the world of ideas of Philinus and Serapion. Thus we cannot compare their motives with those of the Daoists. The two groups—the empiricists and the Daoists—lived under very different conditions. Yet there was nevertheless a parallel.

32 | Manifold Experiences of the World

The era of Hellenism was the first shift in early Western history. The center of power moved. The power structure changed. No center or structure of power has ever lasted longer than three centuries. European medicine had emerged and persisted. But this was not simple. The incessant changes of place and structural framework made it very difficult to find an indisputable model image for a new view of the organism in the human body. Ancient Greek medicine lasted—though the original model image had long since disappeared.

Individual authors continually came up with new thoughts and suggested new hypotheses. They somehow felt that the old ideas no longer corresponded with the reality of their lives. They introduced new teachings into medicine that ensued from their entirely personal model images. Each of these authors lived in a unique environment. Each of these authors had his own, totally specific, subconscious ideas of harmony and crisis, of order and chaos—and how one condition turns into the other. Each of these authors created impulses, drew model images out of his own subconscious experience of the world, formulating new views of the organism.

If many thoughtful people can express their worldviews in totally different ways, then it is a sign that there are many different world experiences! It cannot be expected in such a situation that large groups or parts of the population share one and the same worldview. No one can really sense how things will continue. No common feeling arises. Various people experience the real environment differently. Many see the ideal structure differently—if such ideals exist at all.

This is roughly how we can imagine the time following the decline of the polis democracy. From then on, there was no longer any world experience uniting the majority of society as had been the case during the polis democracy. Therefore, there was also no longer a convincing model image that might have led many to a convincing new image of the organism. Medicine was there, and it claimed to correctly interpret and effectively treat many illnesses. Who could argue with that? Today, too, many illnesses heal, but not necessarily because of treatment. But there were also many who hoped to change the theoretical superstructure. For a long time, no one really managed to create a single, widely accepted new image.

33 | Greek Medicine and Roman Incomprehension

And then the political and cultural center shifted a second time, to Rome. Greek physicians were now attracted to Rome. Power concentrated itself there. An increasingly affluent clientele lived there. Greek physicians brought along their medicine, which they were proud of. And yet they were initially bitterly disappointed. The new medicine, especially the part of it that was interpretation, was not at all convincing to the Romans. Influential orators publicly announced a battle against Greek medicine, even calling it dangerous!

That was quite incomprehensible to Greek physicians. Yet it is comprehensible to us. The Romans never had the model image that lent plausibility to the theories of the Greeks. To the Romans, Greek medicine was a foreign idea with which they could make no associations. The theories themselves, convincing as they had been in Greece, initially had no meaning for the Romans, and even provoked aversion.

Who practiced Greek medicine in Rome? As far as we know, almost only the Greeks! The Roman censor Marcus Porcius Cato (234–149 BC) led anti-Greek opinion. He and his son shared his view of true therapeutics: empiricism and magic. His personal worldview, evidently shared by most Romans, was the model image for this nonmedical therapeutics. He did not share the Greek worldview of the polis democracy that had existed two or three centuries beforehand.

Of course, the Pandora's box had already been opened in Greece, and now many fantasy creations flowed from it into Rome. An author named Asclepiades (first half of the first century BC) followed the impulses of Democritus (ca. 460 BC) and Epicurus (341 BC). So we read in the history books. But why would an author in Rome in the first century BC turn against the humoral doctrine and fall back on the so-called atomistic view? Why did Asclepiades like the idea that material consists of indivisible atoms, dissimilar only in form and arrangement? His opinion was not based on any experimentation—it was a purely mental achievement. Where did he get the impulse? Where did the model image come from? It had nothing to do with reality. Asclepiades gave expression to plausibility.

He may well have been a good observer. Perhaps he pitied the poor patients who had to endure the therapies of the humoral doctrine: bloodletting, emetics, laxatives, sudorific agents. They were drastic. But to most physicians, they seemed unavoidable. They were applied to put the humoral household in order, to restore balance to the mix. But Asclepiades had a different idea: man is made of atoms. The atoms arrange themselves to form pores and pathways, and they move inside these pores. Life consists of this normal movement of atoms in pore pathways. Illness is stasis.

34 | Illness as Stasis

This quite reminds us of the Chinese conception of qi. At the time of Asclepiades, thousands of kilometers to the east, the term also meant fine material particles. They formed matter and they flowed through matter. Free flow is the precondition of life. Stasis is illness. Asclepiades was not influenced by the Chinese. Several centuries beforehand, Democritus and Epicurus had provided him with the first impulse. This is where the puzzle lies. Three centuries before Asclepiades, the ideas that he then took up with some success and passed on to a large following had all been expressed. Why had such a school not formed centuries before? What now gave these ideas the plausibility they needed to convince so many?

Harig called the school of Asclepiades "purely Roman . . . all its important representatives lived and taught in Rome."[30] One might thus assume that they had a common model image. To look for this model image, we must take the situation of Rome as a world power into consideration. Will this help us understand why Asclepiades and his followers came up with the image of the body as being made of "un-joined mass particles"? Why Asclepiades and his followers postulated a "random movement of atoms," and not a regular movement? Why they attributed health to the normality of size, form, and movement of atoms, as well as to the normality of the width and openness of the pores? And why they interpreted illness to be the cessation of normal movement?

It is tempting to answer "yes." At the same time as China was unified, the Roman Empire had annexed an enormous geographic area. The autarchy of the small, familiar polis was forgotten. Now, at exactly the same time as in China, a great empire came into being comprised of varied and increasingly distant units that all had to contribute to the good of the power center. Unlike in China, most of the diverse units remained ethnically and culturally distant.

In ancient China, there were only seven, and then two, states competing for dominance before the unification of empire. They had all been "Chinese" before unification. The teachings of Confucius, Laozi, and other philosophers were already known in all the states that came together after unification. Although the rulers in the capital now presided over many formerly separate territories, the unification of the empire was ultimately a bringing together—albeit through force—of the closely related parts of a preexisting cultural alliance.

35 | Head and Limbs

The expansion of the Roman Empire produced a totally different outcome. Rome annexed lands that previously lay outside of its own cultural inheritance. Ethnic and cultural differences thus remained under the rule of Rome. The dispatching of military and political stakeholders did little to change that. The sense of exchange among equal, individual parts that had emerged in China after unification never came into being in Rome. If anything, there was compulsion to send supplies to the center to support the ever-expanding state structures.

Asclepiades and his followers could thus not have seen things differently. They subconsciously saw the model image in the basic structures of the Roman Empire, and they projected it onto their image of the healthy and sick body. It was the political and economic reality, not the expressive power of the human organism, that was the impulse for their thoughts. It was also what lent those thoughts the plausibility needed for them to be widely accepted. As early as 1928, Owsei Temkin (1902–2002) showed what had played out here.[31] The humoral doctrine is a holistic doctrine; that is to say, in illness, the wrong mixture of humors unavoidably flows throughout the entire body. There can be no partial illness. Illness always affects the entire organism.

The atomic doctrine sees things entirely differently. The doctrine of illness of individual body parts originated from the atomic doctrine. It is not always the entire organism that is sick. And naturally, it is not always the entire organism that must be treated. A localized massage may be sufficient to restimulate a locally disturbed flow of atoms! Where did this impulse come from and where did the plausibility come from? The polis democracy was either completely healthy or completely sick. The Roman Empire could be separately sick in either its head or one of its limbs. If the Roman head was sick, the limbs in the distant regions of the empire were not necessarily also sick. Usually, of course, things go wrong somewhere in one of the limbs. An ordering therapeutic intervention is then needed. The Roman head and all other limbs were hardly affected by that at all—except at the end. By then the head and the limbs were all sick. But that lay in the future, still unimaginable to Asclepiades and his followers.

Once Asclepiades made his thoughts known, other thinkers came and spun them further. Themison of Laodicea (around 50 BC) and others founded the school of the Methodists.[32] They now dominated therapeutics theory. Were their theses more effective than those of competing ideas systems? Certainly not. But they possessed two further advantages: First, the doctrine was simple. Asclepiades was not interested in hidden causes. He wanted nothing to do with anatomy. He was completely opposed to the interpretation of life processes. Second, the therapy was congenial: baths, wine, and water cures. It had to work. It was convincing.

36 | The Rediscovery of Wholeness

Who were the Methodists' main competitors? We observed with fascination that in China the intellectual elite entertained several separate traditions, not only of political philosophy but also of therapeutics. On the one hand, there was the medicine of systematic correspondences of all phenomena, in which we mainly found the world models of the Confucians and the Legalists. This medicine corresponded to structures of the unified empire. On the other hand was the empirical, pharmaceutical tradition of therapeutics that had close links to Daoist political ideals. In ancient Rome, it might seem, the thought of the Methodists sufficed. After all, its theory mirrored the fundamental structural elements of the Roman Empire. But this medicine apparently did not correspond to the worldview of all intellectuals of the time who were interested in solving of the puzzles of the organism. In Rome, too, the elite could not agree on a single system of therapeutics.

The Romans also produced a second influential school: the Pneumatics. Here again, we find a distant echo of the qi that played such a crucial role in the Chinese medicine of systematic correspondences. Or is the simultaneous emphasis on qi in China a distant echo of the Roman Pneumatics? It is indeed strange that the term *qi* first appeared in China shortly after the founding of Stoic philosophy by Zeno of Citium (ca. 336–264 BC) in Greece. From this philosophy, the founder of the Pneumatics, Athenais of Attaleia (ca. 50 BC), borrowed the doctrine of pneuma as the absolute life-giving principle.[33] If the pneuma is altered, illness results. Major alterations lead to death.

Did a model image lend plausibility to this view? We do not know. This doctrine could not have been based on clinical practice. The doctrine of the Pneumatics could not draw its justification from the graphic nature of the organism. No reality in the body could provide a model image. We do not know where it came from. The influences on the thinking of Athenais are even harder to trace than those of Asclepiades and the Methodists. Both were Greeks and used ideas from that heritage. Both were citizens of the Roman Empire, lived primarily in Rome, and were also open to the impression of Roman life.

What constituted the central message of the Pneumatics? The medical historians Aschoff and Diepgen have summarized it as follows: "Under the influence of Stoic philosophy, the Pneumatics bring energy and matter into the closest connection. The common thing, in which both are active simultaneously, is pneuma, belonging simultaneously to heaven and earth, body and soul. Inborn to people and continually renewed through breathing, it penetrates, carried by the blood, all organs and tissues, gives the body vegetative and animalistic life, and also nourishes mental functions. It is the true effective agent in the humors and qualities. Illnesses are ultimately anomalies of pneuma. Its failure causes death."[34] We are used to this by now: pure plausibility. This doctrine was much more sophisticated than the Methodists'. It was also more comprehensive. Asclepiades thought in a purely materialistic way. Athenaios added the spiritual aspect. A century after Asclepiades, we see Athenaios' return to the holistic perspective. There is something, let's call it pneuma, linking the external and the internal, spirit and matter. Was there a new feeling of community here, for which there was no motivation a century beforehand? Perhaps.

37 | To Move the Body to a Statement

Galen is the most famous physician of the Roman Empire. Who knows the names of Asclepiades and Athenaios, other than a few historians of medicine? They were too tied to their time, their teachings were too obviously caught up in temporary plausibility for them to be convincing beyond their own lifespan. But Galen was well known, then as now. One might call him the most successful thinker in all of medicine, at least in the European history of medicine. Galen was Greek and brought the Greek intellectual heritage with him to Rome, in the manner of all his colleagues. He made a name for himself as a successful clinician, and Marcus Aurelius appointed him as his personal physician.

There have surely been many good clinicians in the course of the millennia, but today we barely know anything about the majority of them. A prolific author, Galen's writings were the source of his posthumous fame. He is said to have written at least four hundred texts. On the theoretical level, he was an eclectic. He took impulses from all perspectives known at the time. But even more importantly, he pursued the reasoning of those who saw holes in the veil of plausibility. With great resoluteness, he set out to observe reality. He rigorously pursued reality as the basis of his medical interpretations.

But what reality? Did we not agree that the body, and with it the organism, possesses little expressive power? After a long break of four or five centuries, Galen resumed the long line of those who attempted—and still attempt—to prompt the organism to express itself. For this, one must get close to the organism. Questions must be asked. The body is only capable of answering the questions that have been asked. And someone asking questions must, of course, have something in mind. He who looks at the body to find his own constructed image confirmed remains distant from reality even if he is in contact with it. It seems that Galen was also burdened with his own preconceptions as he posed questions to the body and the organism. Yet he did not completely screen out reality. He was relatively open to what the body offered as reality in response to his experiments and his questions.

Ingo Wilhelm Müller summarizes Galen's encounter with reality quite nicely:

> In numerous details, he enriched knowledge, particularly with good descriptions of the muscles, bones, and joints. He was the first to differentiate clearly between nerve, tendon, and ligament, and he refuted the idea that nerves are hollow. . . . In numerous simple but well-conceived animal experiments he proved . . . the automaticity of the heart and the generation of breathing movements by muscle power, and differentiated voluntary and involuntary muscles. By clamping an artery in two places and cutting it open in between, he showed that arteries contain blood, not air. He closed off the urethra and found that this stops the flow of urine into the bladder . . . he cut through nerves and parts of the spinal cord at various places, and demonstrated functional relationship between the brain, spinal cord and peripheral nerves through the resulting paresis. Pressure on the exposed heart was ineffectual on mental function, whereas pressure on the brain induced stupor. In the age-old debate on the location of the soul, this was the first experimental argument for the brain as the source of emotional and mental powers.[35]

That was indeed impressive. Never before, and not for another millennium into the future, was reality approached so closely. Not until the sixteenth century did other researchers forge ahead with comparable abandon, seeking the view of the body without always being shackled by the chains of longstanding model images. Much of what Galen discovered is still considered to be true and valid. However, the knowledge of anatomical details and simple functional processes in the body that Galen discovered through his experiments did not lead him to the holistic view of the organism that we might adopt today. Müller even refers to a "theoretical edifice that appears nightmarish to the modern researcher, speculation inhibiting progress." Yet, along with other historians, he is right to ask how it could have lasted for so many centuries.

38 | Galen of Pergamon: Collector in All Worlds

We need not occupy ourselves here with the details of this theoretical edifice, which can be found in the respective works on the history of medicine. Galen worked out the insights from his experiments using set pieces from earlier attempts at interpretations, some of them dating back to the Greek era, and added his own conclusions. For example, there are his views on the source, flow, and function of blood. Galen did not come up with the idea of a great circulation that some authors had postulated earlier in China. He could see no such circulation in the body. Impulses from his living environment clearly did not suffice to inspire this idea. Galen was also an Aristotelian philosopher. He knew Aristotle's teachings on the circulations in nature. He was unable to bring together the circulation in nature and the flow of blood in the body. An impulse was missing. In his time, it could have only arisen from his living environment—and it seems that there was no such impulse.

Galen had received a comprehensive education in Greek philosophy and medicine before he went to Rome at about thirty years of age. That is to say, his worldview was that of Greece, but of a Greece that had already long been part of the Roman Empire. Before his departure to Rome, Galen had treated gladiators in Pergamon. His pronounced interest in the anatomical details of the body can be traced back to that experience. But what about the interpretive part of his medicine, physiology, and pharmacology? Here, it hardly seems possible to separate the individual impulses from each other. Only the fact that he was the prototype of the eclectic gives us a clue. In a cultural environment that could hardly offer a clear mark to a wanderer between the Greek and the Roman worlds, eclecticism is the most obvious path. As the Roman Empire incorporated things from the various cultures, Galen likewise collected ideas here and there and put them all together in his own system.

In his system, pharmacy found a theoretical grounding for the first time. Galen created the first pharmacology in the history of medicine. This should not be taken for granted. The pharmaceutical substances made from natural plants, roots, rinds, blossoms, and leaves, not to mention certain animal products, already had a long history behind them. But so far, no one had made any efforts to bring the knowledge of the therapeutic effects of the natural drugs into harmony with the four humors doctrine that had already been passed down for six or seven centuries.

Do we remember our astonishment upon learning that in Chinese antiquity, the scientific doctrine of systematic correspondences was initially not applied to the explanation of the effects of pharmaceutical drugs? It seems it was no different in European antiquity—but in a totally different context!

39 | Europe's Ancient Pharmacology

What was the worldview, what were the interests that had prevented pharmaceutics from being consistently incorporated into the four humors doctrine in Greece and in the Roman era before Galen? For China, it is not difficult to recognize. We have already discussed it sufficiently. And for European antiquity? We have not yet posed this question and must leave it unanswered for now. It is a fact that Galen the eclectic integrated pharmaceutical therapeutics, hitherto external to medicine, into medical therapeutics. To rephrase this: Galen expanded medicine with theoretically founded pharmaceutics. He drew on the ideas of the four humors doctrine and developed it into a comprehensive pathology of the humors, the so-called humoral pathology. He drew on the knowledge of the effects of medications and created pharmacology—the scientifically based study of the effects of medicinal substances on the human organism.

This was no easy task, even if we grant that the results can in no way compete with the pharmacological knowledge available today. Galen's task was to unite the four parts of the four elements doctrine with the seventeen different then-known effects of pharmaceutical substances. The result was very convincing, on both the cognitive and the aesthetic level. It united the plausibility of theory with the reality of the properties of the substances. That a pharmaceutical drug can produce a warming or cooling feeling in the body is a reality that several people can experience independently of each other. Also, the ability of a substance to influence digestion, break open an ulcer, or increase urine flow is reality. Plausibility comes with the pharmacological interpretation: Why does a substance stimulate urine flow? Interpretation may be based on the doctrine of the four humors, conceived from the view of reality and the logic of the available theory.

Galen's contribution was as brilliant as it was simple. As had already been known for a long time, in human beings there is a mixture of the four humors: phlegm, blood, yellow bile, and black bile. However, the perfect balance is never reached, so that each person has his own, more or less unbalanced, mixture—his idiosyncrasy—and with it, his own character. In the natural substances, it is similar. In each, the four basic qualities—hot, cold, wet, and dry—may be present in a different mixture. They are supplemented by two additional qualities: coarse and fine. Thus, every effect can be definitively explained, including if the effect is quick or slow, or if it occurs superficially or deep within the organism.

At this point, we should again turn to China. At the very same time as Galen there lived a man named Zhang Ji (ca. 200 AD). We have already encountered him as the author who tried to connect the scientific doctrine of systematic correspondences (i.e., the theories of yin-yang and the five agents) on the one hand, and pharmaceutics on the other hand. He was not only a contemporary of Galen; he also had similar ideas. He was the first known author in China who tried to incorporate pharmaceutics into scientifically based medicine, that is, to develop a first pharmacology. Admittedly, the result was rudimentary. The time in China was not yet ripe for such developments. We shall soon see when and why the time did become ripe. But this much can already be revealed here: the consistent pharmacology that Galen created in Rome found its first parallel in China in the twelfth to fourteenth centuries.

40 | The Wheel of Progress Turns No More

And Galen's effect on history? His fame was first described in late antiquity by Oribasius, a physician-author in the fourth century AD. Oribasius and other physician-authors of the following two centuries had no further creative impulses; it seems that the Roman Empire had arrived at the end of its cultural creativity, along with the era of Greek development aid workers. There nothing was left to do but study the legacy and, for the contemporaries who still had an interest in such knowledge, to condense it into ever smaller, more compact compendiums.

The medicine that had developed so impressively from the pre-Socratic philosophers of nature—with Hippocrates leading the way, followed by many more or less renowned authors of ancient Greece and the Hellenistic period, and finally culminating in the work of Galen in the Roman Empire—and which had gone through such a remarkable development between reality and plausibility now lost its importance. The knowledge of reality was hardly of any use. A new theoretical edifice was not in view. The plausibility of the theories also seemed to be lost.

Didn't the "cataclysmic unrests" that shook the empire in its last centuries show that order was merely an illusion? Was it time to believe in demons again? How much power did people have over their fate? Were the Christians right? Was all being and nonbeing, all existence, attributable to their one God? To many highly educated people, nonmedical therapeutics once again seemed more convincing than medicine. The situation was muddled. No one could give a final or comprehensive answer. There was no feeling of departure into a new era as there had been in China when the empire was first unified after traumatic centuries of war or as there had been in Greek antiquity with the new structures of the polis and democratic ideals.

Now, at the end of the Roman Empire, dissolution was everywhere. The Roman educated class retreated to the new elite stronghold of Constantinople. The proletariat stayed. Rome became barren, with a doomsday-like atmosphere. Nothing new was created. As some isolated thinkers clung to the now rather old medicine, the view of the body stayed right where Galen had left it: humoral pathology, the doctrine of the significance and the right mixture of the four humors, phlegm, blood, black bile, and yellow bile. The changing excretions, colorings, and smells of the body in healthy and in sick days provided adequate proof that these teachings corresponded with reality. Enemas and bloodletting, emetics and sweating may have helped many people and corroborated the truth of this doctrine. However, the momentum of the theoretical insight came to a standstill; the wheel of progress in interpretation no longer turned.

It is not as if, as one occasionally reads, Galen dominated European medicine for fifteen hundred years. It is true that Galen was the most important figure in the rediscovery of the ancient medicine in the Late Middle Ages and the early modern age. The Renaissance was indeed a new beginning! In this era, the enthusiasm and spirit of departure could be felt everywhere! However, this departure was initially much more indefinite than at the times when a new medicine was created in Chinese and Greek antiquity. There was initially no new image—neither of a new social environment nor of the body. These things would not appear for a very long time. Initially, European intellectuals again concerned themselves with redrawing the picture of antiquity. It was amazing how much they already knew back then! Aristotle's and other great philosophers' theories were brought back to awareness.

None of the many authors toward the end of the Middle Ages made any great breakthroughs; they all puttered around with various questions about details. For want of a better leading thinker, Europe initially oriented itself toward the man whose texts were generally available and who seemed to be the only one, at least until the sixteenth century, who had mastered the Herculean and now barely imaginable task of dissecting the body and looking into the organism. The therapeutic doctrine was now, as then, simple and manageable: emptying of excessive humors via bloodletting and laxatives, emesis, sweating, and similar techniques. Occasionally, an operative intervention such as removal of bladder stones. But that was a mere craft and had nothing to do with interpretive medicine. We will discuss the European Middle Ages and the Renaissance in more detail.

41 | Constancy and Discontinuity of Structures

And in China? How did things continue there after antiquity? The Han dynasty existed at almost the same time as the Roman Empire. It fell, however, in the early third century; the Roman Empire likewise tottered worryingly, but did not collapse into the two halves of Western Rome and Eastern Rome until the fourth century. The last Western Roman emperor was deposed in the year 476. If we compare the fates of the two empires, we see two entirely different developments. In China, the Han empire broke up, but the resulting individual parts basically continued the same culture that had served as the foundation for the Han dynasty. This would continue until the beginning of the twentieth century.

It is true that foreign rulers came to China. Northern people of the steppe, nomads, repeatedly managed to conquer a China that was no longer militarily fit and to set up their own dynasties. But each time, the foreign rulers eventually became even more Chinese than the Chinese themselves—they adapted to the high Chinese culture. Thus, Chinese history is full of manifold political dramas. Rulers and dynasties came and went, yet the cultural basis always remained the same. Confucianism, Daoism, and Buddhism, in all their more or less profound reformulations and conceptual extensions, always oriented themselves toward their roots.

Though the great canon of ancient literature was often reinterpreted by contemporaries, it remained the same in its essence. We must keep this in mind as we compare and seek to understand medicine and especially the interplay of plausibility and reality in the two medical cultures of China and Europe. In China, not only did the cultural ground from which every era drew its own meaning remain the same, the ruling system also remained essentially the same: an empire and its bureaucracy. Of course, there were various interpretations of this. The Mongolian rule from the thirteenth into the fourteenth century and the following Ming (1368–1644) and Qing dynasties (1644–1912) were markedly more autocratic than earlier eras. But the ideal and fundamental structure always remained the same. And, importantly, through the intimate familiarity of every educated person with the history and the origins of the state, the old ideals and basic structures were in everybody's mind. A stable and lasting education system ensured that it remained that way.

We must be aware of this constancy in China if we want to understand its history of medicine. We must also be aware of this constancy if we draw comparisons with Europe. Was there ever an era in European history that maintained the same cultural foundation for more than three or four centuries? Was there ever an era that preserved the same ruling structures for more than three or four centuries? No, there was not. And often European intellectuals could also simultaneously observe different ruling structures in nearby, neighboring societies. The consequences for medicine should not surprise us.

If the image that people—thoughtful, intelligent people—make of the body and of the organism, in interpretation and from seeing the organism itself, is influenced by real or ideal social conditions, then European medicine would have to develop totally differently from Chinese medicine. If ideas about how the harmony of the social organism is safeguarded or disturbed and how to avoid social crisis and uprisings affect one's ideas about health and the explanation of illness, then European medicine since antiquity must have gone through much more intensive and even radical changes than Chinese medicine.

And yet there are the almost unfathomable parallels. What did we just say? The momentum of theoretical insight came to a halt; the wheel of progress in interpretation stopped turning. This refers to the difficult time at the end of the Roman Empire and in the first half of the Middle Ages, up to the scholastic era. During this time, no new ideas enriched European medicine. In therapeutics overall, there were a few innovations—but only in the nonmedical part of therapeutics.

42 | Arabian Interlude

Arabian authors had just as astonishingly and single-mindedly incorporated the knowledge of Greco-Roman antiquity, organized it, and added a few of their own thoughts here and there. There was not a major change on the theoretical level, since these authors came from the outside. The view of the organism they found in this medicine had no counterpart in their living environment. How could they have given it new impulses? A few marginal contributions were achieved solely on the basis of internal logic. This medicine was so foreign to the thinking and worldview of the Muslims that the guardians of the faith soon advised abandoning it and returning to the nonmedical therapeutics oriented toward the sayings of the prophet.

That should no longer surprise us. It was not the clinical effectiveness, not the internal logic of medicine that possessed a comprehensive power of persuasion. Neither was it the extremely impressive texts that Arab authors wrote about this medicine. Did it not seem that Albucasis, Razes, and the rest of them claimed the medicine of Greco-Roman antiquity for themselves and made it their own? It only seemed that way. It was individual scholars who felt attracted by the variety and the depth of thought in the innumerable writings of ancient authors. But they still remained mere individual scholars, who would never be able to convince their native culture, especially those scholars who represented the original, religious Muslim worldview of this culture. The clinical practice of the crusaders was also unconvincing in the long run. It was simply too primitive compared to the procedures they already knew themselves. Thus there was, also in this respect, no reason at all to look up to the European healing culture in the long term. Arabs again disappeared from the stage of European medicine.

Where in China do we find the parallel to these events in Europe? Wasn't the founding of the Tang dynasty the beginning of one of the most fruitful eras in all of Chinese history? From 618 to the start of the tenth century—almost exactly three centuries to the year, the Tang era brought back together what had broken apart following the end of the Han dynasty. But not only that. Possibly no other of the great, long-lived dynasties of imperial China shone as brilliantly as the Tang dynasty, on the inside as well as on the outside. No other civilization could be as proud of such intensive relations with foreign lands and cultures as the Tang. The great cities constituted fascinating depositories of many peoples and religions. Trade brought wares from distant non-Chinese regions to the kingdom. Nestorian Christians, Jews, Manicheans, and many other groups more were attracted to China to share in the wealth.

43 | The Tang Era: Cultural Diversity, Conceptual Vacuum

And in medicine? Nothing happened at all. No new ideas were added to the theoretical foundations that were handed down from the Han era.

Pharmaceutical drugs from the rest of the world came via long trade routes to China. For the first time, a pharmaceutical book was compiled at the request of a government and published in 659. It listed 850 individual drugs—many of them from distant lands. An example is theriac, the wonder drug that Mithridates once developed as protection against poisoning and that, in changing compositions, played an important role in European pharmacy until the nineteenth century.

Indians and Nestorians from Persia also came and introduced eye treatments hitherto unknown in China, among them the cataract operation. As varied as such manifold contacts with foreign therapeutics were, they had no influence on Chinese theory. Sun Simiao (581–ca. 682), the man we might rank as the most influential Chinese physician and author of all time, was an exceedingly, comprehensively educated man and simultaneously a competent clinician. In his writings, we find traces of Indian Ayurveda and the humors doctrine of the distant Mediterranean. Buddhist ideas were also familiar to him. Wouldn't he have been the man to further develop medical concepts?

A good question. A naïve question. Why should he have wanted to develop it further? It was working well. He had collected thousands of prescriptions for all possible illnesses. The prescriptions were obviously effective; the fame of his therapeutic abilities reached all the way to the emperor's court. He was a favored guest. Some illnesses ended with death, irrespective of all physicians' efforts. After all, there are limits to the physician's art. A better pharmaceutics must be sought; more effective prescriptions must be compiled. But theory? The theory was consistent. Nothing had changed that might have threatened its plausibility. On the contrary, the entire Tang era was proof enough that the old concepts worked. Everything was going as well as could be. Who was interested in deviant thoughts about harmony and crisis? There was no crisis. Thus we find the astonishing simultaneity of developments in Europe and China. With respect to the view of the body, we can now ascertain what happened in both cultural areas—the radiant China of the Tang and the darkened Europe of the Middle Ages. The momentum of interest in theoretical insight came to a standstill; the wheel of progress in interpretation stopped turning.

Yet let us reexamine this closely. Was there really no noticeable crisis in the Tang era? Apparently not for most people, who enjoyed an eventful life. But something else was being hinted at. For some Confucians, the situation even appeared threatening. They nervously followed the political tendencies, were vigilant, and eventually concluded that Confucianism, hitherto the basis for safeguarding the moral foundations and bureaucratic administration of the empire, was showing signs of weakness. Daoism and the foreign teachings of Buddhism had found increasing numbers of followers and even entered into official ceremonies!

Han Yu (768–824), a poet and official, raised his voice in warning. The Buddhist cult of the relics was his point of departure. He used this to underline his criticism of the increasing influence of Indian religion. He paid dearly for this—almost with his life. Appeals by his friends reduced his sentence to mere banishment. Li Ao (d. 844), a philosopher, was more clever. He wrote a medical text. In this text, he hid his political suggestions for reforming Confucianism. The doctrine was clearly missing some attractive content that had diverted followers to Daoism and Buddhism. Confucianism had never sought to occupy itself with nature; it emphasized the morality of human relationships. Confucianism also offered no metaphysics, no warmth of understanding, no mercy, no forgiveness. Buddhism offered these things.

For his text, Li Ao chose a plant that he could be sure was not yet described in pharmaceutical books: knotgrass. To this plant, he linked a story about an old, infertile man who falls asleep drunk in the wilderness and awakes the next morning to see two intertwining stalks of a strange plant he has never seen before. In the story, loaded with innuendo, the impotent drunk stands for Confucianism, and the two plants are Daoism and Buddhism. The drunk follows the advice of his friends and drinks a carefully-strained extract of the two plants, and—lo and behold!—soon fathers many sons. His survival is assured.

Yet in 974, some physicians missed the underlying message of the story. They took the recommendation at face value, and added it to a pharmaceutics book. Since then, Chinese medicine has considered knotgrass an important pharmaceutical ingredient that can make the old turn young and turn white hair black. After all, Li Ao was a well-known philosopher.

Who would mistrust his recommendation? The plausibility of the effects of knotgrass has survived in Chinese pharmacy until today.

44 | Changes in the Song Era

The political message of the knotgrass story may have been lost on many, but Li Ao's recommendations nevertheless became official policy about three centuries later. The Chinese themselves refer to it as the Song doctrine. Philosophers of the Song era had the initiative to tackle the renewal of Confucianism that Li Ao had not dared to speak of openly. And they had a prescription for the problems of Confucianism. They opened the door to intensive occupation with nature, thought up cosmologies to link the world of men with the natural universe, and created a metaphysics to successfully compete with the Buddhist doctrine: all men are brothers.[36]

At the center of these thinkers stood Zhang Zai (1020–1077), his two nephews Cheng Hao (1032–1085) and Cheng Yi (1033–1107), their teacher Zhou Dunyi (1017–1073), and finally the great philosopher Zhu Xi (1130–1200), who synthesized the individual thoughts into an impressive whole. Zhang Zai confronted Buddhism by convincingly arguing that the material world is real, not imagined. Reviving Han era ideas, he wrote that finely distributed matter, qi, can form anything and disperse again. Since we are all made of qi, he concluded, we are all connected with each another—and obligated to each other. The Cheng brothers came to the conclusion that an abstract structural pattern underlies all real phenomena. Every thing and every person has a certain structure (li). To understand the essence of a thing or person, it is necessary to study this basic structure. The structures of all people are connected. And all people are also connected with the universe.

Zhu Xi cited these ideas, as well as the global model of Zhou Dunyi. He showed that to understand people and nature, both qi and li must be considered. Li is always the same; qi can change and become impure. This explains, for example, differences in character among people. It also demonstrates where education and upbringing must start. The important thing is that two goals were reached with this philosophy: the necessity of being kind to and having sympathy for one another. An ingenious solution to the problem of the formerly lacking metaphysics. Concern for nature was now just as justified as concern for people. The hitherto separated worlds came together as equals and a new view of the world emerged.

But there was more. A non-Chinese people conquered north China. The Jurchens, nomads of the steppe, began their invasion in 1126. The centuries-long emigration to the south increased again. Endless streams of refugees left the northern lands. Populations in the cities swelled to millions. Economic centers were now concentrated in the south. Many things changed, not only in political philosophy, but also in very concrete, everyday politics and economy. "The rapidly-growing complexity of the economic structures influenced trade and transportation above all. Numerous new inland waterways were built, and a whole shipbuilding industry developed in Shensi [Shaanxi], Kiangsi [Jiangxi], and Chekiang [Zhejiang]. As on the emperor's canal alone, total rice shipments were twice what they had been in the Tang era, coastal shipping was also increasing in economic significance, and for the first time there was noteworthy Chinese overseas trade, hitherto mainly left to Arabic and Persian traders. . . . The upswing of the money economy and of trade are intimately connected."[37] And so on.

By the Song era, things were looking up again, despite the loss of land in the north. Trade blossomed. Regional centers formed around certain product lines and became so specialized that they needed things from more distant regions. A feeling of mutual dependence intensified. No one could do everything themselves. But together, they could do everything. Was there not a similar feeling shortly after the first unification of the kingdom in the late third and early second century? And perhaps an even more intense one now?

45 | The Authority of Distant Antiquity

A tension-filled situation emerged. The philosophers had created a new world view: Neo-Confucianism. This view of human society and of nature offered itself as a new model image for medicine. Did we not already observe such a triple jump in antiquity? First the new social order, then the new view of nature, and finally the new view of the body. Neo-Confucianism inevitably affected medicine. But the effects remained superficial. They joined the Confucian-Legalistic medicine with the pharmacy that had been established under Daoism. We shall take a closer look at this later. For now, we will ask why there were no more profound changes in the direct realm of medicine, that is, in the interpretation of the organism and the structures of the body.

After all, the basic structures stayed the same. Empire remains empire. Bureaucracy remains bureaucracy. Why should a new body image, a new understanding of the organism, have emerged? In the Song era, the image from the classic of the Yellow Thearch in the Han era was once again clearly reaffirmed: regions are connected and goods are exchanged on many routes. That was still true. It was now even more the case than in previous centuries. The general validity of the old teachings was accepted. We even read of a new minor excursion into anatomical reality. In the eleventh century, an autopsy of criminals is documented. What result was to be expected? At any rate, it did not change people's view of the organism.

Since the fourteenth century, images of the body have been printed in China. They depict a rough morphology with the organs that were known since antiquity. These pictures of the body can possibly be traced back to anatomical pictures from far earlier centuries. They could possibly be traced back to the dissection in the eleventh century. The important thing is this: they were never changed. Not until the nineteenth century. The body had been looked into once or twice. What was seen was drawn as accurately as possible. That was enough. It seemed to concur with the descriptions in the ancient texts. It was also known what happened in these organs. The physical organism does not make powerful statements. It is the social organism that supplies data for interpretation.

The new data offered clues, but not a revolution. This was China, not Europe. Confucianism was expanded and newly interpreted, yet progress always cited the supposed or real authorities of distant antiquity that these new views were made to resemble. Nothing new was desired. New things had to come in old cloaks. Only then were they acceptable.

Physicians luckily found a real authority from the Han era to whom they could trace their innovations. The innovations were not only due to the changed social philosophy. Seemingly marginal structural changes may also have made a contribution.

46 | Zhang Ji's Belated Honors

For example, in the eleventh century, the Chinese government opened state apothecaries and published prescription books shortly thereafter. These were set up so that the educated patient could find his symptoms indexed in a table with the indications for the prescriptions. He could then go to an apothecary and buy the medicine. Taking it would bring the desired cure. This was a wonderful thing. To Confucians concerned about morality, the profession of the physician was burdensome. People, in particular children, were obligated to help the sick. Employed physicians made a profit from this. Who could be sure of their motives? This was to be put to an end. The professional physician was superfluous— the path of the patient now led directly to the apothecary.

Physicians saw this—or at least one, Zhu Zhenheng (1281–1358), did. He recorded his thoughts on the matter, which are still available to us today. He used sarcasm to make a comparison. Someone who takes a prescription because it healed an illness in the past has about the same chance at success as someone who goes out to buy a thoroughbred with a picture book in his hand. Or as someone whose sword fell overboard in the middle of a lake and has no time to look for it today, but will return to the same place tomorrow. To mark the searching place, he carves a notch into the side of the boat where the sword fell into the water. Zhu Zhenheng's point is that this is hopeless.

Zhang Ji, who in 200 AD had taken first steps to create a scientific pharmacology and was then largely ignored for a thousand years, now arrived at unhoped-for honors. We can see a slight parallel to Galen in Europe. In China, Zhang Ji, like Galen, was elevated to the role model of the new era—and at the same time! Zhang Ji was the ancient authority whose ideas could be continued from where he had left off. Had he not started what was now to be completed? The joining of Confucian theory and Daoist nature studies—pharmacy? Many authors felt inspired to complete this work. They created all kinds of models of how to integrate pharmacy into the doctrines of yin-yang and the five agents. Why only now? Why more than a thousand years after all the necessary ingredients for this mixture had been made available by the thinkers of the Han era?

It is baffling that this simple task had not been attempted much earlier. It was only one thousand years after both Galen and Zhang Ji had attempted very similar undertakings that Chinese intellectuals finally got around to doing what they had long failed to do. And why? Clinical necessity, perhaps? Certainly not. Perhaps because new insights into the processes in the organism offered new possibilities to better explain the effects of pharmaceutics in this same organism? Certainly not. No, it was simply the transference of political philosophy onto medical philosophy.

47 | Chinese Pharmacology

The Chinese authors who created the new pharmacology starting in the eleventh and twelfth centuries were not narrow-minded physicians who focused solely on the human body's suffering and remained isolated from history, politics, and the ideas of their philosophers. Narrow-minded specialists, as even today, may have been the majority. But they were not the thoughtful ones, not those who come up with innovations. Innovative physicians subconsciously implemented the political program of Neo-Confucianism in medicine. As the political philosophy of the Neo-Confucians restored the comprehensive validity of Confucianism and incorporated themes hitherto reserved for Daoism, they produced, for the first time, the comprehensive validity of the doctrines of yin-yang and the five agents by applying these to the explanation of the effects of the pharmaceutics in the body. That they also happened to serve the political interests of professionally practicing physicians is a nice arabesque. Political philosophy and professional physicians' politics permitted the origins of pharmacology.

Pharmacology and professional politics? Pharmacology and professional political interests? What political advantages did physicians have from pharmacology? The state supported the apothecaries. It guided patients directly to apothecaries. It even introduced the legal obligation to give a pharmaceutical brand name to new mass-produced preparations, which was intended to limit the flow of counterfeits into the market. With pharmacology, physicians hoped to have created a strong basis for winning patients back. The goal was to lead patients to the physician first.

It is not unusual in China for doctors to offer a diagnosis for free and to earn their living from the sale of pharmaceutics. For this, patients first need to see a physician instead of going directly to an apothecary. This was the task of pharmacology. It gave physicians the knowledge of where and how pharmaceutics worked in the body. Pharmacists only knew the symptoms and sold prescriptions that appeared to be effective against those symptoms. The physicians, however, wanted to control the dispensing of pharmaceuticals. For that, they came up with a brilliant new formulation of the old game "We see something you don't see!" Unfortunately, we no longer know who invented this game. If we did know, we would still be honoring him or her today. So how did this game work?

48 | The Diagnosis Game

Brilliance is always connected to simple solutions. The simple solution here was the following: the same symptom in two sick people does not necessarily mean that both have the same illness. Or: two sick people with different symptoms do not necessarily have different illnesses. Thus, it is important to look past the external symptoms of a sick person, to "look inside" and diagnose the underlying disease there. Each disease is different. A disease does not necessarily always express itself with the same symptom. Only the physician can "see" the details of the individual illness inside the body. Physicians "see" something that the pharmacist and patients do not see.

Thus, the preparation of the physicians' game went like this: First, they created a pharmacology. That is to say, they finally incorporated the properties of pharmaceutics into the same theoretical framework that had already included the body functions for over a thousand years. Then, they claimed for the physician an exclusive ability to determine the individual condition of the patient by looking into the body through diagnosis. Finally, they claimed the ability to compile great and effective prescriptions for the condition of each individual patient through the linking of their diagnostic and pharmacologic knowledge.

With that, the physicians had created a basis for argumentation that allowed them complete freedom of action. Let us think about the consequences of this new game of "we see something you don't see." Only physicians could recognize people's internal conditions. One would stand or sit next to a patient, look at the patient's face, listen to the patient's voice, ask how he or she is feeling, and take a pulse. Then, with a serious demeanor, one would make a prognosis: a yin illness in the kidney. No one could verify it. Objective patterns of interpretation hardly existed. Not even today. Every physician in Chinese traditional medicine can make up his own story. No one else can disprove or refute it. The literature of that era and the times that follow shows that anyone can play this game as he sees fit.

49 | The Physician as the Pharmacist's Employee

Were they successful? Yes and no. Patients continued to go directly to the pharmacist. A saying even arose that turned around rules of the game. The saying goes: "The pharmacist has two eyes: with the one he sees the illnesses, and with the other, suitable pharmaceutics. The physician has only one eye. He sees only the illnesses, and knows no pharmaceutics. The patient is fully blind. He knows neither his illnesses nor the suitable drugs." Since then, there have been doctors in China who sit as employees in the offices of the pharmacists. Almost every apothecary in China—in both rural and urban areas—has employed physicians, if the pharmacist is not active as a physician. Since patients go directly to the apothecary anyway, it is natural that physicians also locate themselves there. The apothecary has physicians diagnose the patients and write out prescriptions.

This is not what Zhu Zhenheng and others had in mind when they thought up the game with the various individual diseases. But working in the apothecary as an employee of the pharmacist, examining patients and writing prescriptions was still better than having no patients at all. Of course, we do not want to exaggerate here. There were also plenty of successful physicians who established themselves so that that they could work independently.

Have we just discussed a pharmacology? Indeed we have. But this statement could be misunderstood if the emphasis were on a single "a." Here, "a pharmacology" means that people thought about how pharmaceutics could be incorporated into the doctrines of yin-yang and the five agents, to explain their effects in the organism. Yet this is not the same as saying that *a single* pharmacology was created. Many different solutions to this problem were presented. One might also say that once the basic rules of the game were established, various creative people went about applying these basic rules as they saw fit. Thus it could happen that what one author judged to be a yin quality was determined by another to be a yang quality. Many different models appeared on the scene. There were no objective standards for organizing the classification. Who could have made an impartial decision based on facts? Nobody.

Reality looked different to every author. But that did not matter. In the foreground stood the subconscious compulsion to create an argument in which the illnesses and pharmaceutical drugs comprised a net that could catch patients. Thus, each author created his own net. Because others likewise created nets to catch patients, everyone criticized each others' arguments and tried to tangle them up so that only their own net would emerge as tear-proof. A standard net that all fishermen might have used was never made. Why? It seems they all worked equally well. Each of them produced a satisfactory catch. That was the most important thing. Someone made a net out of the idea that people suffered from too much heat influence. This net caught just as many as the idea that all illnesses were caused by digestive problems. The second physician was also right—especially since he lived at a time of war and famine, when such ideas can really gain plausibility. Didn't they emerge from the reality of life?

50 | Relighting the Torch of European Antiquity

Once again, this was an exciting, dynamic era. So many new ideas! But no one wanted to admit—or even better—no one *could* admit, that the ideas were new. Everyone claimed to be reviving the true tradition of antiquity that had long been transmitted underground. How did Confucius describe himself? Not as a creator, but as a transmitter. This was the model. Whoever cared about his reputation and sought success presented his ideas not as a new birth, but as the rebirth of an ancient knowledge that had long been ignored due to adverse circumstances. Rebirth? That has a familiar ring—it sounds like the Renaissance. And with that, we are back in Europe.

Was there not also, at the western edge of the Eurasian continent, a simultaneous rebirth of ancient knowledge that adverse circumstances had long prevented from emerging? The Renaissance in Europe occurred under entirely different preconditions, and was not a rebirth in the literal sense of something dead being revitalized. An interest in the ancients, or even engaging in dialogue with them—as Petrarch did with Cicero—does not bring them back to life. Yet it was also a rescuing of ancient authors and their knowledge from obscurity. An astonishing parallel.

Let us again consider the developments of the Early Middle Ages in Europe. Here are some of the catch phrases that two of the scholars best-acquainted with this era, Gerhard Baader and Gundolf Keil, have found for it: "Reception of generally inferior sources of ancient medicine . . . language of a vulgar caliber . . . no power of abstraction . . . content often thinned down, occasionally of Byzantine origin . . . supplemented by folk medicine elements . . . application of a primitive medical practice."[38]

That does not exactly sound like admiration of the achievements of the scholars of the time. Perhaps the Early Middle Ages really were such a pathetic era. But there are other voices, too. They indicate that at the

time, other signposts were followed than in the preceding and following centuries. Jacob Burckhardt called the Middle Ages an era in which
"life was more colorful and rich than we can even imagine today."[39] The
remaining historical sources are unclear. Who can judge? Of course,
there is little to report in our area of interest. That would not change
until the eleventh and twelfth centuries, when the attempt at a reacquisition of ancient medicine began.

We speak of a reacquisition, or, better yet, the attempt at reacquisition. This choice of words is intentional. May we—as if anticipating
the Renaissance—also speak of a rebirth? Rebirth: something that once
existed comes back into the world and is born again. Can medicine ever
be reborn, go through a renaissance? To be reborn, first something has to
have died. By all appearances, ancient medicine had indeed passed away
in late antiquity and the Early Middle Ages. Yet medicine had not totally
disappeared. Texts survived here and there. The Arabs, as we have seen,
were interested in them for a while. Then there was the renewed interest
of Christian Europe. But—and this is the most important point—there
was no rebirth.

It is easy to understand why medieval medicine narrowed ancient
medicine down to only the fraction that might suffice to treat common
afflictions. Theory became uninteresting. The environment that might
have allowed it to develop further, or even to maintain the greatness it
had once achieved, was missing. Its practice—as the Muslim observers
of the crusaders reported—was anything but sophisticated. Why the
change in the eleventh century? In retrospect, we do not know why the
change occurred. There is no satisfactory explanation. One could list
the impulses for the so-called European Renaissance in Italy from about
1350. There were so many changes in the political landscape there that no
one is surprised it affected thinking in art, literature, architecture, and
science. But in therapeutics, in the eleventh century?

In the eleventh century, there was a medical school in Salerno, in
southern Italy. Was this a spontaneous development? Did the impulse
come from the Arabs? Was there perhaps a surviving enclave of ancient
culture that revived for some reason? We do know that southern Italy
was settled mainly by Greeks well into the fourteenth century. In Sal-

erno, Greek Orthodox and Roman Catholic clergymen celebrated mass together until the early fourteenth century.[40] Somewhat later, a medical school in Montpellier was added, perhaps not by chance. Montpellier was situated near the Arab-Islamic region in neighboring Spain. However, that alone does not explain why there was renewed interest there for the old knowledge. Perhaps a look at Toledo will help.

Won back by the Christians in the year 1085, Toledo was geographically even closer to Arab-Islamic culture. In 1135, the archbishop founded a translation center there where translators were highly active until 1284. This led Dag Nikolaus Hasse to ask:

> But what were the political interests of the archbishop of Toledo? It is suspected (by Richard Lemay, for example), that in the translations, the archbishop saw a welcome means in the fight against the Islamic enemy, intellectual munitions for the refutation of "heresy." Yet the true enemies of the archbishop in the twelfth century were not the Muslim armies in the South, but the archbishops of Braga and Santiago de Compostela, embittered opponents of the dominance of Toledo as the spiritual metropolis on the Iberian peninsula. . . . The translators Gerhard of Cremona and Dominicus Gundissalinus belonged to the cathedral chapter of Toledo and thus to that political elite that actively and with some success aspired to (pre)dominance over all the Christians of Spain.[41]

This dominance also implied a leading role in the recovery of ancient wisdom. "Happy," wrote Gundissalinus, "was the early era that produced so many wise men who lit up the darkness of the world like stars. The sciences that they founded are left as torches to light up the ignorance of our minds."[42] Relighting the torches with this Christian light seemed desirable—whoever managed this could claim leadership, power, and influence. This may have been the motive for policy. For those eager to learn, the main wish was to renew Aristotle's worldview and put it to use in the Christian context. Medical texts soon followed. In the twelfth century, the remaining original Greek sources were then translated into the now conventional Latin. In southern Italy in the twelfth and thirteenth centuries, Greeks were still present as mediators. Hebrew documents were also available for evaluation.

The quality of the Latin versions must have been dreadful enough to make one's hair stand on end. The translators simply proceeded word by word, often without any feeling for the content of the original message. The simultaneous attempts to transfer Latin texts into vernacular versions were no different. Baader and Keil described this as follows: "It is hardly necessary to point out that the translators struggled with syntax problems and often got shipwrecked in their attempt to translate hypotactic Latin into vernacular language, resulting in a chaos of incorrect associations and anacolutha that run throughout the texts."[43]

This was the manner of reacquisition of the once sophisticated ancient inheritance. In Latin, a word-for-word transfer; in the vernacular, an often meaningless string of individual statements. On both levels, there was the imperfection of a terminology that still had to be created. It was difficult to read into these texts. It must have been a strong incentive that motivated this search and supported the various centers. The court of Anjou also participated. When Robert I ascended to the throne in 1309, he promoted an even larger translation project than his ancestors; it continued even until his death in the year 1343. What motivated this? What advantages did it have for the initiators of this development? So far, we have no good explanation.

51 | The Primacy of the Practical

Much of what happened at that time in Southern Europe, France, and eventually also Central Europe reminds us of China—yet the parallels are not profound. The comparison is limited to the rough dating of events. China and Europe both looked back to antiquity, but with totally different preconditions. In China, something new was attempted that had the appearance of the old. Europe initially had nothing new in mind. The thirst for knowledge, fed by obscure sources, concerned itself with the reacquisition of ancient knowledge, true to the original.

The fate of pharmacy is also noteworthy here. The profession of pharmacist did not originate in Europe until the twelfth century. Pharmacists were responsible for producing medications. Thus, pharmacy branched off from medicine as its own discipline. This is the exact opposite of the simultaneous development in China. There, medicine incorporated pharmacy. Here, the rulers separated pharmacy from medicine. There, physicians were employees, dependents of the pharmacist. Here, pharmacy remained subject to physicians. When Emperor Frederick II declared the first medical ordinances in 1231, he made physicians warders over the pharmacists. In the oldest German apothecaries' ordinance, the ordinance of Basel in 1271, pharmacists were even forbidden to issue any medication at all without a physician's prescription. Zhu Zhenheng could only dream of that!

The nature of the new healing that originated in the High and Late Middle Ages is also noteworthy. Practical concerns predominated. Prescription books were written and widely disseminated. The celebrated *Antidotarium Nicolai* originated as early as the second half of the twelfth century. It replaced the older, seemingly useless *Antidotarius magnus*, whose author had still closely followed the now distant Greek models.[44] The arrangement of the prescriptions in the *Antidotarium Nicolai* did not follow indication groups or a theoretical classification of illnesses, but rather a simple morphologic scheme, from the head down.

Known and loved alongside the drug descriptions and prescription books were also the so-called *regimina sanitatis*—instructions on how to live a healthy life. Salerno was the first to develop a good reputation for these. The educational text on "how to maintain good health" originated between 1100 and 1150. The content of these texts was down to earth. Diet and hygiene rules were based on either ancient or Arab traditions. The goal was to educate people about the optimal lifestyle. Apparently, not everyone shared the conviction of devout Christians that the body is relatively unimportant and what counts is the soul.

A new sentiment possibly arose in some places. It seemed enticing to pay less attention to saving souls than to the well-being of the body. So one took a new look at the obvious: air, eating and drinking, movement and rest, sleep and waking, excretions and secretions, and moods. Clothing, dwelling, and sexual intercourse were also worthy of attention. These were clearly visible aspects of human existence. No profound theory was needed to recognize that a disturbance of these aspects made people sick. Just like the old Silesian saying: too much or too little is always a problem! The Greeks spoke of the *medèn agàn*, the Chinese of the doctrine of the mean. Admittedly, even the practical Salernitans wanted a bit of explanation. They drew on the elements, the four humors, and the soul.

Orientation toward reality was sought in another area as well. In imperial China, as we just mentioned, only a single autopsy has ever been documented, in the eleventh century. It had no discernable impact on the view of the organism. In Europe, things were entirely different. It seems that since Galen, no one had even dissected an animal, let alone a human, to study its structure and function. There is no evidence that the Church officially prohibited dissection. Yet the Christian environment did not encourage such activities either; on the contrary, numerous statements from Church voices opposed such studies.

Theological misgivings obstructed the quest for knowledge. The question of resurrection had not been unequivocally solved. Was it the whole body, or only a bone, or perhaps only the spiritual element? Opinions were divided. Toward the end of the thirteenth century, Mondino de Luzzi (ca. 1270–1326) of Bologna wrote his renowned textbook *Anatomia mundini*. Surely he had looked at one or another corpse himself. But he did not see much. Galen's great anatomical work had not been translated yet. Mondino relied on a physiological text of Galen's in which the ancient author also included much anatomical knowledge. This was the seed of a new beginning.

Mondino worked in Bologna. The focus there was on law. The desire to solve a poisoning murder led to the first forensic autopsy in Bologna, in 1302. It is possible that even a few years earlier, a corpse or two had been opened for medical study. Padua followed Bologna's example in 1341, Perugia in 1348, Montpellier in 1376, and Florence in 1388. In Spain, the first recorded autopsy was in 1391; in Vienna it was not until 1404. But nevertheless, an avalanche had started that would not be halted. We shall return to this.

So much practical healing. So many new efforts to understand the reality of the body. Yet this was not a revival of ancient medicine. Can we already speak of a new medicine? It is missing an important thing that is important to us, the element that allows medical healing to emerge from nonmedical healing. Medicine, we agreed at the outset, is the part of healing that has cast off everything numinous and trusts only in the laws of nature to explain the organism and to derive from this understanding the necessary measures for the prevention and treatment of illness. Did such a medicine exist in the eleventh, twelfth, or thirteenth century? No. Clearly it did not, at least not as a living body of theory and practice.

In Arabic and Greek texts, ancient knowledge—what we recognize as medicine in the true sense—lay hidden. Inadequate translations of these texts into Latin and vernacular languages hardly made it suitable for revival. People were concerned with experiential wisdom about balance in waking and sleeping, in eating and drinking, and so on. And there were countless prescriptions and many roots, leaves, blossoms, and stems that were believed to be helpful for all kinds of indispositions and complaints. Early anatomy initially served only to confirm the statements of Galen, but not to scrutinize his theoretical knowledge, much less develop it further. All of this was not medicine; it was therapeutics without medicine.

52 | The Variety of Therapeutics

Therapeutics was also understood in the sense of salvation. It was not only that a practical, experience-based, nonmedical healing emerged into the foreground. The influence of the Christian worldview had already been fostering a religious healing for centuries. However, Church officials disagreed as to whether people should trust in faith and prayer alone, or if God had put healing herbs into the world for humans to cleverly use to their advantage.

Amid such uncertainty, it is not surprising that astrological, magical, and demonological therapeutics found wide dissemination. A case of worms, for example, could be treated with medications, with appeals to God, or with simple exorcism. Oak leaves were a beloved remedy, since it had been known since pre-Christian times that the oak was the tree favored by the gods. Faithful Christians knew that Satan fears the oak. The authors of the popular rules of the month, documented since at least the eleventh century, recorded some entirely practical suggestions. For example: In January, it is always healthy to eat warm food.[45] Such knowledge was connected with astrological findings.

We could fill many pages with lists of the ideas and practices that marked the therapeutics of the time. The relics cult, for example, is worthy of further attention. The Christian worldview lent it plausibility for many people. But where was the reality if, for example, a monastery marketed cough syrup throughout Europe made by dipping a martyr's hair into water and selling the thus ennobled liquid? The therapeutics of the time was endlessly rich and conceptually varied. It was just not medical.

Medicine requires science. Science requires knowledge of the laws of nature. Why would people in the eleventh, twelfth, or thirteenth century have concerned themselves primarily with such questions? The situation was not at all as clear as it had been during the Greek polis democracy. It must have been a confusing time, the path ahead anything but straightforward. With the decline of the Roman Empire, the persuasiveness of the idea of laws of nature apparently also declined. Was there a reason to resurrect them again to the forefront of the worldview, of the view of the body? Not yet. There were more urgent tasks. The Scholastics came to the forefront with their attempt to unite Christian teachings and ancient philosophy.

But in retrospect, on another level it is hardly surprising that therapeutics was so manifold and medicine so limited. Let us forget the lack of a science for a moment. Also lacking was the model image for a clear view of the body. The anatomists conducted autopsies. But with their view into the corpse, they sought the confirmation of the meager knowledge taken by Mondino from an anatomically insignificant text of Galen's and from his own experience. It did not enter the anatomists' minds to go past this knowledge. Nothing in their environment inspired them to do that.

Let us take another look at the point of departure of the new medicine in antiquity. The situation in the Greek cultural domain led the way: the development of the polis democracy. The ideal (and in some respects even the real) structure of the societal organism offered insights into the structure of the body. The initial situation in China was similar. From the sociopolitical upheavals and social philosophies of the fourth to second centuries BC, two opposing traditions emerged, each with its own view of the body. Yet the two basic directions of thought were clear and understandable.

We now turn to the so-called High and Late Middle Ages. The involved regions stretched from Spain in the west to Byzantium in the east, from Central Europe in the north to southern Italy in the south. Do we need to examine each of the many political and cultural, social and economic peculiarities of the landscapes in this region? Any list here would be incomplete. Was there anything that might have influenced the intellectuals who were active in this region with similar clarity and persuasiveness as had been the case in Greece and China? That is hardly conceivable. What worldview, what ideas or order did people in Constantinople, still Eastern Rome, share with Greeks in southern Italy and Sicily, with the Islamic Moors in Spain, or with the crusaders in Central Europe?

The worldview and the ideas of order that united at least some people were those of the Church. Yet their kingdom was of a different world. The Church preferred to focus on the hereafter. For many scholars, the body was a mere receptacle; for some, even a burdensome receptacle for what was truly valuable: the soul. In any case, there was no impulse from the Church to learn about the body. Its kingdom offered no model image, so no new view arose.

53 | Which Model Image for a New Medicine?

As the knowledge of antiquity gradually flowed back into the minds of Europeans, it was completely detached from its original cultural and social context. It had to stand on its own. This is no easy task. Can a philosophical knowledge of nature that developed in a polis democracy simply be transferred onto the clerical and feudal structures of the Middle Ages? Can the thoughts of Aristotle, Plato, or Plotinus simply be brought into the intellectual world of the French nobility or the awakening bourgeoisie of Italian city-states? Didn't the cities have totally different interests and ideas of order from the kings or the Church rulers? All of this did not fit together. It was not made to fit together. Everything had to be painstakingly reassembled. So many thinkers had a worldview to offer. So many suggestions on how the world should be formed.

Yet initially, there was no formation worth mentioning at all. Perhaps this is not only an impression that emerges in retrospect. Perhaps contemporaries already felt the decline and chaos in the unordered variety of impressions. After all, so many worlds were involved! Added to the variety of European and Mediterranean lands were now impressions of travels to Asia, Africa, and, following 1492, the "New World." Where were these people, animals, and plants described that one could now marvel at? But something else was also new: the first "Hundred Years' War" between England and France, from 1338 to 1453. Two rival popes at the same time, from 1378 to 1417. The plague starting in 1348—and the loss of a quarter of Europe's population.

People had a real go at each other.

> Seldom were so many rulers murdered or deposed in such a short length of time. A Neapolitan tyrant stuffed his dead opponents with straw, dressed the mummies in their own clothes and displayed them in a gallery . . . and yet there was also another side to this era. European cities flourished again despite all the wars and ongoing plagues. In Italy, the first banks were established; thriving wholesale trade spread across Europe and all the way to Asia . . . wealthy princes and citizens became patrons and founded the first private libraries and galleries of the modern age.[46]

Indeed, it was confusing. Who could have recognized a clear path there?

Giovanni Pico Della Mirandola (1463–1494), the Italian humanist and philosopher, included Persian, orpheistic, and kabbalistic teachings in his personal syncretism. This was fascinating and very erudite. But no more than a handful of aesthetes followed him. This was true about the others as well—in the preceding two or three centuries, and again in the following ones. A variety of suggestions were presented by more or less great minds, based on their own impressions and with their respective backgrounds of basically random acquisition of various materials from the established cultural heritage. Initially, no one managed any great breakthrough. That would have required a basic sentiment that united a great number of thoughtful people. Things had not yet progressed this far in the eleventh to the early fifteenth century.

For medicine, a convincing model image was missing of the real and ideal structures of society, a model image that could have lent plausibility to a new view of nature and then, in a third step, to a new view of the structures of the body and the organism. The many attempts and suggestions by the intellectual world speak for themselves. Never was it as clear as in the two or three centuries from the end of the thirteenth to the sixteenth century: countless professors and students, among them surely many of the most talented and most intelligent, looked into countless corpses. They carefully cut out heart, lungs, kidneys, tendons, muscles, and whatever else they found. They held it all up and looked at it from all sides. And the result? There was none. The body itself possesses no power of expression.

54 | The Real Heritage of Antiquity

For over two centuries, the organism had a chance to explain itself. But it did not, because it could not. It is speechless and does not reveal its interior. Externalities, yes. But not the interior, the connections, the functions. The organism only reveals these in response to concrete questions. But to ask such a question, one must know what one is looking for. This was lacking from the thirteenth to the sixteenth century. Professors and their students were not looking for anything in particular, and therefore failed to ask any suitable questions. The organism thus produced no answers and revealed only its externalities—the heart, lungs, kidneys, vein valves, and so on. Otherwise it remained silent.

Without science and without an image of the organism, how could a medicine develop? The work of Abbess Hildegard von Bingen (1098–1179) has met with fascination until the present day. In her text "Causes and Treatment of Illnesses," she suggests something that one might expect to have been greatly persuasive in the Christian West. She linked surviving elements of the ancient humoral and elements doctrines with fundamental ideas of Christian theology. Why she singled out phlegm as the most important cause of illness is unknown. In her understanding of the world, she attributed afflictions of the human body caused by phlegm to sin before God. Her therapeutic suggestions are similarly wide ranging, linking the theological/spiritual with ancient pharmaceutical heritage and folk therapeutics knowledge. However, that was not

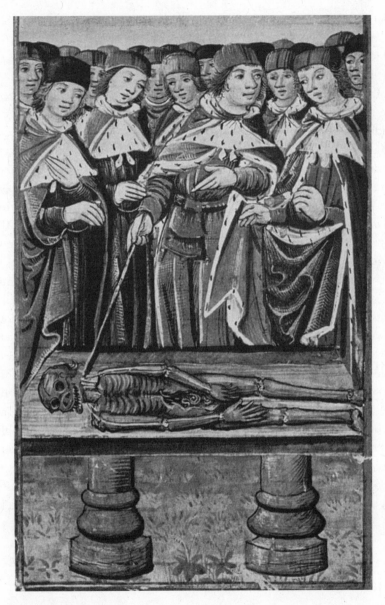

Figure 2. Instructions in Anatomy. Miniature, ca. 1465. Reprinted with kind permission of Glasgow University Library, Department of Special Collections.

enough. Hildegard von Bingen appealed to some contemporaries. She still appeals to people, even at the beginning of the twenty-first century. But she did not plant the seed of the new medicine.

It is clear that old preexisting set pieces served, because of the lack of other knowledge, as the foundation for suggestions for a comprehensive therapeutics. A new medicine could not yet develop because the fundamentals were missing: science and a convincing societal model image. But here lay the opportunity for Europe! Everything that had lent plausibility for the creation of the first medicine was missing—and since there was no plausibility because no model images were available, there was nothing else to do but study reality. But what is the use of studying the organs of the body if they remain silent? There is indeed a use: the exact knowledge of the body's anatomical details serves a corrective to theory, which is only accountable to plausibility.

This is the real, lasting legacy of Western medicine. It is the only aspect of ancient medicine that was carried over into the new medicine of the second millennium. Here lies the lasting, fundamental difference between Western medicine and Chinese medicine: the self-sufficient polis democracy was possibly responsible for the relative disinterest in large-scale, extensive relationships. From the beginning, the interest in the substrate was stronger in Western medicine than in Chinese medicine. In ancient Greek medicine, this feature was still balanced by theory. Theory was primary from the outset. It seemed so natural, so probable, that reality never came into question as a corrective. The ancient Greeks were keen observers. Their portrayals of the morphological details of the body and the progression of illnesses are unparalleled in antiquity. However, theory was draped like an opaque veil over reality. The Greeks looked at so much, and yet they saw so little.

55 | Galenism as Trade in Antiques

That was different now. There was no longer any theory, only set pieces that formed no coherent whole. Everyone had his or her own interpretation. The only thing that appeared to be the same to everyone was the reality of the external appearance of the body and organs. At first, organs that had been cut out of the body were simply gawked at. "Ahs" and "ohs" likely resounded in the crowds of spectators (occasionally numbering in the hundreds) as the dissectors removed another organ and held it up high for edification. But then came Johannes Winther of Andernach's (1487–1574) translation of the great anatomical works of Galen, and soon afterward, the breakthrough. Vesalius (1514–1564) is remembered as the symbol of this breakthrough, though he was not the only person involved. The others, however, are now known only to historians. What happened? In Europe, and only in Europe, an active, indeed aggressive, entrance into reality was achieved, completely detached from any living theory. It was an amazing process that received only passing enthusiasm. But it lasted long enough to lay the foundation for a much more resilient tendency.

One might object that Galen's knowledge experienced a thorough reacquisition and was further developed to the extent that some historians— above all the great Owsei Temkin—even spoke of "Galenism"![47] Was that not enough theory to cloud the eyes of the dissectors? For many, this may have been the case. The Parisian anatomist Jacques Dubois, named Sylvius (1478–1555), the teacher of Vesalius, was one of them. He had accepted the new knowledge of the vein valves from younger anatomists. But apart from that, he saw the interior of the body only as Galen had presented it over a millennium beforehand. Sylvius trusted the statements of the ancient texts more than his own eyes. There have always been people who cling to antiques, polish them up a bit, and keep them for their everyday life. They may delay progress a bit here and there, but not for long. Sylvius had brusque words for Vesalius, calling him a monster who poisoned the air. Vesalius was also conditioned by Galenic theory. But he and many others of the time no longer let themselves be totally blinded by Galen's veil. They saw holes in the veil, and they looked through these holes in a consistent way, without needing a model image. Vesalius's discovery that Galen's anatomical descriptions were based on the interior of animals, not humans, helped to strengthen their research.

Reality was honored. "Progress in anatomy in the early modern age was slow; the distancing from Galenic anatomy was gradual."[48] This is expressed carefully. A tendency was born. The path was cleared for completely new things. However, the path initially lacked a goal. There was no guiding image and certainly no model image. That is the astonishing thing. Even without a guiding image, the anatomists forged ahead into reality. They looked at it and saw something. To the extent that additional details of reality were constantly revealing themselves, it became ever clearer that Galenism was a trade in antiques. Aesthetically pleasing, no doubt. Those who attempted to breathe new life into the old theory were certainly not untalented. But their attempts amounted to nothing more than dated nostalgia.

This should not surprise us. In the twenty-first century, too, there are groups with anachronistic world views. Yet molecular biology and gene research have taken their course. So it was also in the fifteenth and sixteenth century, when Berengario da Carpi (1460–1530), Nicolo Massa (1485–1569), Charles Estienne (1505–1564), Giovanni Battista Canano (1515–1579), and Andreas Vesalius (1515/6–1564) published their views. They were not totally blinded by the copies and reproductions of Galenism. They were not without prejudice, but they were still impartial enough to explore the details of the body's reality without being led astray by a prefabricated theory. The plausibility of the ancient teachings faded because its model image had long since disappeared. A new image was not in sight, and this created the opportunity for reality to be discovered.

56 | Integration and Reductionism in the Song Dynasty

In the late Song era, Chinese intellectuals had a clear, new image before their eyes. Neo-Confucianism and existing social and economic structures were simultaneously a confirmation of the old and an impulse for something new. Yet many people in China soon found themselves without orientation in history, like their contemporaries in distant Europe. Is that not strange? Chinese and Greek antiquity were incomparable in politics, society, and economy. In spite of these differences, both civilizations had produced a medicine for the first time. In both, the patterns of society were applied to nature and then to the explanation of the organism. The simultaneous periods of the Early Middle Ages in Europe and the Tang dynasty in China were also incomparable in politics, society, and economy. Regardless of these differences, both remained theoretically unfruitful to the same extent. In the following epoch, starting with the eleventh century, the High and Late Middle Ages of Europe and the Song, Jin, and Yuan eras of China were incomparable in politics, society, and economy. Regardless of the differences in cause and effect, we can now, in retrospect, observe the attempt at a new beginning in both ancient civilizations. And the eras that followed? It was no different. Who called the shots?

In the Song dynasty, the old three-step repeated itself: first came the new formation of society—ideal and real. The change was not as profound as at the beginning of the period of imperial rule. Nor was it comparable to the upheavals in Europe. But nevertheless, the expansion to include fields hitherto reserved for Daoists and Buddhists went along with new economic data. An expanded worldview developed on the foundation of traditions, which were now over a millennia old. Next came the second step: a new connection with nature. Everyone, including Confucian scholars, was urged to examine it for themselves. Finally, the third step: a changed medicine. This was the medicine of the Song era.

This was a very complex medicine, initially visible in a simple integrative approach—found in the great prescription collection, *Shengji zonglu* (1111–1117). All published knowledge, regardless of its heritage, was compiled, including instructions from the common people. Twenty thousand prescriptions were gathered together, medical healing unproblematically united with nonmedical therapeutics. Long chapters about the natural laws of systematic correspondences were placed between long chapters of countless apotropaic formulas from the realm of demonology. Astrology was also included. Were there no longer any guidelines? Effectiveness was all that counted. The new pharmacology was integrative, though of course on a more demanding level. It brought medicine and pharmaceutics together. The old theories of systematic correspondences of all things now incorporated, for the first time, the explanation of the effects of pharmaceutical drugs in the organism.

But there was also an opposing tendency that emerged in the search for the causes of illness. Most authors of the time maintained the reductionism that traced suffering to a single main cause—heat, cold, or gastrointestinal upset. Where did the plausibility come from for this narrowing of perspective, even as the view was simultaneously expanded? Perhaps we can see the contradictory developments on the socioeconomic level: the expansion of the scope of Confucianism's worldview, alongside the economic specialization of the individual regions. Specialized knowledge and skills also seemed unavoidable to some reformers. The old ideal of the comprehensively educated scholar, who could competently handle all administrative tasks, began to falter. In the eleventh century, Wang Anshi wanted to train specialists for the legal, financial, and military systems, for geography, and for medicine. His reforms did not remain valid for long. But the ideas survived. The break from universalism could no longer be reversed.

What started in medicine under the Song continued under the Jurchens of the Jin dynasty and the Mongols of the Yuan dynasty. That was the dynamic: every idea system develops once it has had the chance to establish itself. This dynamic guaranteed survival and continuation, even if the original environment that gave the impulses, the model image, no longer existed. Schools exist. Teachers educate students. The image survives, purely on its own. It needs no further external stimulation. Its plausibility now stems from its own internal logic. Reality—whether a construct or really existing—was now a minor consideration.

Indeed, the Mongols soon let the model image of the Song era fade away. In the year 1260, Kublai Khan declared himself ruler of a northern Chinese region; two decades later, in 1280, the Song dynasty disappeared. Great efforts had been made during the Song era to confer new, ever more comprehensive validity onto Confucian social teachings, and such innovations flowed into Neo-Confucianism. But then came the Jurchen invasion, which pushed Song society into the south. The Jurchens were followed by the Mongols—uncouth, but strong on horseback and in battle—who conquered all of China. Gone was the dream of reawakening the greatness of the Han dynasty.

Mongolian rule over China lasted until 1368. The rulers took Chinese names and tried to create a dynasty similar to those of their Chinese predecessors. There was a high degree of continuity, yet something was missing: access to the intellectual world of the conquered. Agriculture, trade, and, more importantly, the administration of such a large area by means of an efficient apparatus of officials—all this remained foreign to the nomads from the steppe. The Chinese upper class arranged themselves with the invaders as best they could, but it did not go well. Soon, the economy declined. Initially, the anger of the impoverished was directed at everyone "up there." Then came the nationalistic motive of defending China against the foreigners. The Chinese upper class eventually sided with the rebels. Hardly a hundred years later, a Chinese ruler once again sat on the emperor's throne. The country was saved. So at least, it seemed.

57 | The New Freedom to Expand Knowledge

The new dynasty called itself the Ming, or "the enlightened," but the illumination was clearly not very profound. The Ming rulers found themselves in a unique situation—all political interests within the country were balanced against each other. This was an opportunity for the rulers. It was the opportunity to establish absolutistic rule! Never before had a Chinese emperor reached comparable power. The Confucian officials remained stripped of power, as under the Mongols. They quarreled among themselves in excessive group struggles and, through the well-aimed interventions of the government, became increasingly marginal.

In keeping with their origins as an uprising "from below," the Ming rulers implemented democratic reforms. Down with civil-service examinations! An elite instrument for suppression of the lower social classes! Several education systems have been destroyed with this argument. Not that state examinations could be totally abolished. But they could be made so simple that everyone would pass. We are familiar with this from our own recent history. The conservative officials' class in China was also introduced to it. They also were astonished to learn that practical skills were now more important than an elite literary education. We are familiar with this, too.

The rulers endorsed Neo-Confucianism, but the method of learning was mechanical: memorize the texts and then recite them in an exam. Don't waste time on the contents. Studying became a mere formality. It had no influence, at least no lasting influence on later thinking and action. People complained that class differences became blurred. Even slaves could now get an education, even if it was usually only a sham education. The result was fascinating: those at the bottom entered the world of those at the top. Those at the top came into contact with the views of those at the bottom!

Things started to move. In the Song era, several physicians and observers of nature had used the new freedom to "investigate things and expand knowledge." They arrived at completely different results. Everyone had a different conclusion as to why people get sick. Everyone proclaimed his own prescription for preventing or healing illness. This individualization of opinions increased during the Ming era and gained such momentum that it retained its dynamism even into the succeeding "pure" dynasty, the Qing.

The Ming dynasty flourished for about a hundred years. Then mismanagement set in. Natural catastrophes increasingly impoverished the population. Uprisings started at the beginning of the seventeenth century— again, from the bottom up. Again, peoples from the northern steppe—this time the Manchus—took advantage of the situation. But they were better prepared than the Mongols. They had already set up a practice Chinese state outside the gates of China. That was convincing to the Chinese upper class! The Manchus were allowed in. Better conservative foreign rulers in power than Chinese social revolutionaries. Thus began the Qing dynasty in the year 1636.

58 | Healing the State, Healing the Organism

Though the Manchus were conquerors and foreign rulers, they wanted and were gradually able to adopt the refined lifestyle of the conquered. Yet the braided queue hairstyle forced on the ethnic Chinese was a daily reminder: after the Mongols and the Ming interlude, China had once again fallen victim to foreign invaders from the north. At first glance, the structures were the same as they had always been. In fact, for over a century, they flourished as never before. During the reigns of Emperor Kangxi (r. 1662–1723) and Emperor Qianlong (r. 1736–1796), the country flourished in every respect. It seemed Chinese. And yet it was not. The taint of foreign rule always enveloped the Manchus. This intensified as things began to decline following Emperor Qianlong.

Many Chinese asked what had gone wrong. Did they have the right political philosophy? The Song doctrines seemed increasingly suspect. Surely they were the reason for the inability of the Chinese to rule their own empire. Gu Yanwu (1613–1682) raised his widely respected voice: Empty theorizing has robbed our officials of the ability to assess political realities and to protect our empire from disaster. The fatal problem is the influence of Daoism and Buddhism on Confucianism. Many scholars agreed. But what had there been before the Song era? Could it be revived in the present?

Everyone who cared about the well-being of the country felt a sense of responsibility. Where in the past did the cultural strength of China lie? What would the future hold? The structures had been constant for one and a half millennia. But the spirit permeating these structures no longer fit. So the search began. So many scholars, so many solutions. And medicine? It led the way. Since the political philosophers did not yet possess the courage to articulate themselves, they found expression in medical allegories. Healing for the state was expressed as healing for the organism. To reverse what had newly come along in the Song era! Pharmacology! Nothing but meaningless theory. Suddenly one saw what had not been seen before: the unsuitability of the theories to explain the reality of drug effects. Thus, back to reality, substances, and visible effects. No further knowledge was needed. The empiricists of the Roman Empire would have felt right at home in this environment.

59 | Trapped in the Cage of Tradition

The search for the path out of misery was difficult. Here again, we find simultaneity with Europe. Despite all the contradictions of the concrete situations. So many observers, so many insights. Everyone saw something different. Everyone tried to find a convincing way out of the perplexity. And yet all remained trapped in the cage of tradition. The cage was made of the doctrines of yin-yang and the five agents, of the systematic correspondences of all things. Some observers of nature and physicians even caught new prisoners in this cage: demons. As it had been with pharmaceutics, now it was with the inclusion of demons: a blueprint had existed since antiquity. Only now, after one and a half millennia, did it find it broad acceptance. Do demons exist or not? That was the fundamental question. Some argued that everything was imagined. Others claimed that it was a reality of our environment. They saw red, green, yellow, black, and white demons—linked with the heart, liver, spleen, kidneys, and lungs. This was a last attempt to extend the plausibility of the theory.

Independently of this, there certainly was a whole lot of new knowledge, free from interpretation and taken from reality. In the middle of the sixteenth century, Li Shizhen (1518–1593) wrote his summary of the study of Chinese pharmaceutical drugs: the *Bencao gang mu*. Many observations lay hidden in this huge work, which has never been adequately translated into a Western language. It contains knowledge of botany, hygiene, and other areas that Europe only developed very much later. For example, the insistence on disinfecting the bed linens and clothing of the sick. In China, there were always clever observers. They noted their observations. The old theories were unsuited to explain everything. Simple observation, without interpretation, remained. For example: eyes worsen if one constantly reads or writes by artificial light, or if one carves fine ivory for a long time. Why? It simply is so. Reality.

Some observers of nature looked around outside of people. What makes people sick? That still had to be thought out. Cold, heat, dampness, the wrong food, overexertion, wind—these had been known for ages. From 1641 to 1644, an epidemic swept through the northeastern provinces of China. Wu Youxing was a sharp observer. Patients had headaches, backaches, and pain in the hips and eyes. They suffered from deafness, vomiting, fever, the inability to urinate, stomachaches, and bloating. He had the sick take saltpeter along with other medications and was successful in treating them. Someone had obviously found the right thing. Someone was very close to reality. Dr. Hermann Hager's *Handbook of Pharmaceutical Practice* of 1885 records the effects of saltpeter: "It is an antibacterial, cooling, thirst-reducing and diuretic remedy." Congratulations, Mr. Wu Youxing!

Responsible for the epidemic, according to Wu Youxing, was an "especially terrible fine particle," *liqi.* A hundred years before Wu Youxing, Fracastoro in Europe had suspected *animalculi* as the cause of sicknesses. He thought of them as being just as small as Wu Youxing's "especially terrible fine particle"—a vapor similar to the "miasmas" that Pettenkofer named as the cholera pathogen in the late nineteenth century, while others already spoke of a "contagion." No one had seen either the miasma or—before Robert Koch—the contagion.

Something exists in our environment. That was indubitable—in China as in Europe. No demons, no ghosts. Miniscule life forms, Fracastoro's *animalculi,* or purely and simply pathogenic particles, Wu Youxing's *liqi.* They force their way into the body and make the person sick, not necessarily immediately. Wu Youxing recognized that in some people, the pathogen initially sleeps for a while. This we now refer to as the incubation time. Only subsequently does the illness break out and require treatment. When in the nineteenth century, following prolonged and stubborn resistance by respected experts, the pathogen theory was finally declared a scientific fact, it was not staggeringly new to the Chinese. Somehow, people had long since known about it: demons, *liqi,* bacteria—only the names changed. The idea was the same. Plausibility met reality. Again: Congratulations, Mr. Wu Youxing!

Some observers looked downward in the search for reality. Was there anything to be learned from the common people? Printed texts were the foundation of medical theory and practice. But only the theory and practice of a small minority was actually based on these texts. Ninety percent of the population of China, or perhaps even more, knew nothing about these texts and followed entirely different thoughts in response to illness. Hardly anyone paid attention to this knowledge. Hardly anyone wanted to learn anything from the common people. Especially since there was no medicine to be found there. Therapeutics yes, but still a highly unorthodox one. At best, it was a collection of experience. At worst, it was disgusting.

For example: One sticks a needle into the body and it breaks off. What should be done to remove it? In peasant knowledge, an answer is found. Take a living rat, skin it and remove the skull, spoon out the living, pulsating brain and stroke it on the spot where the needle disappeared into the skin. The needle will resurface on its own. Not all scholars shied away from the encounter with such knowledge. One such exception was Zhao Xuemin (ca. 1730–1805). He published the knowledge of an itinerant physician. Not everything: some things seemed absolutely obscene to him. But he offered the remainder to his readers. A rare view into a different world of healing.

60 | Xu Dachun, Giovanni Morgagni, and Intra-abdominal Abscesses

Some observers looked with interest into the interior of the human without opening the body. They let their thoughts wander into the organism. What meaning did the kidneys have? How important is the heart? They found the answer in old texts. There, some things were written about the organs. This had to be interpreted correctly. Perhaps stomach, spleen, and kidneys were the central organs? And is there really a fire in the body? After all, sometimes the temperature goes up, and sometimes it goes down. The answer was sought in old texts—and found there, too. That was the problem. As Benjamin Hobson (1816–1873), an English physician who was active as a missionary in China for two decades and published the first Chinese-language multivolume work on Western medicine and science between 1850 and 1858, wrote in the preface: In China, perfect knowledge is sought in the texts of the past, whereas in Europe it is sought in the research of reality, in the future.[49]

The Chinese diagrams of the interior of the body that were shown to Benjamin Hobson were not that bad. They were based on models from the twelfth to fifteenth century. Why should the body have changed since then? Everything could be seen in the diagrams: the lungs at the top, the heart underneath, then the spleen. On the side: the gall bladder, then the liver. Even deeper, the small intestine, large intestine, kidneys, and so on. These pictures were everywhere, always in the frontal view. After all, there was nothing missing. All the organs that were described in the texts of antiquity were visible in these diagrams. Things were different in Europe. There, antiquity had made a sort of comeback in Scholasticism, but eventually remained foreign. Humanism focused on *humaniora*. Nothing was excluded from the study of "human matters." In this environment, Vesalius developed—led by the search for something new, by curiosity.

Late, too late, one or another observer in China also took out a loan on the future. In the year 1771, a famous physician and author died: Xu Dachun (b. 1683). In the same year, 1771, the famous physician and author Giovanni Morgagni (b. 1682) died in Italy. If only the two had met! That would have been a stimulating discussion. Chinese and Western medicine as opposites? An invention of the late twentieth century. Xu Dachun and Morgagni would have been surprised. So much in common! Xu Dachun would even have laughed. He was scholar with a sense of humor. As the author of an essay "about intra-abdominal abscesses," he would have been ideally prepared for a meeting with Giovanni Morgagni, the great initiator of morphological pathology of his time.

Intra-abdominal abscesses have nothing in common with "Traditional Chinese Medicine." They were knowledge and reality. Xu Dachun encountered this reality often. In the late twentieth century, "Traditional Chinese Medicine" was discussed in many Western countries. Xu Dachun was overlooked. Some people go into raptures over the "noncausal thinking" in Chinese medicine. Xu Dachun wrote something they should take to heart. Put briefly: "Where illness develops, there must be a cause!"[50] Period. It is sad to bid farewell to this clever man. Therefore, we shall include one more quote. "Facing illness is like facing a hostile enemy. You must be familiar with the foreign land and also with your own land. Then you will be able to attack the enemy on many fronts and avoid having to mourn your losses later."[51] The comparison is a bit militaristic, but that was commonplace at the time. The important thing is that, with this comparison, Xu Dachun demanded an exact knowledge of the territory where wars take place. And this territory is, of course, the human body. Morgagni would have been enthused about this. It is truly sad that we can only bring the two together now, on paper.

Wang Qingren (1768–1831), a physician, took up the impulses of Xu Dachun—consciously or subconsciously—and would probably be remembered as a Chinese Vesalius, if he had been helped by Jan Steen van Kalkar. He saw what many others surely saw. But he was the only one who understood what he saw. Day in, day out, his path led him over a field of corpses. The corpses of children lay destroyed by stray dogs and natural decay. Wang was initially disgusted. He covered his nose, mouth, and eyes. But then he took a closer look and saw astonishing things. Things that looked a lot different than the diagrams in the ancient texts. He was certainly not the only one who walked through the field of corpses. But he was the only one whose curiosity was piqued. Now he looked even more closely, conducted intensive studies, and one day was certain: the ancient texts and the diagrams from the fourteenth century were far from reality. That would have to change.

It did change. But for that, other impulses besides his were needed—as penetrating as the descriptions in his book were. He was not the first to direct people's gaze to the reality of the interior of the body. Western anatomical books had already arrived in China and questioned the old diagrams from the fourteenth century, but hardly raised any interest. "Seeing the big picture" remained the catch phrase until the end. Not to divide and endlessly subdivide. How could the essence of things ever be recognized that way? First, the big picture—the entire structure of the imperial period, and with it the Confucian web of relationships—had to collapse. Only then could the individual's view of the human be free and meaningful.

61 | Acupuncturists, Barbers, and Masseurs

Oh yes, there was acupuncture, too! If we have not discussed it up to now, it is because in China it had fallen into obscurity during this time period. This was already hinted at in 1500. Wang Ji, a renowned physician and author, was surprised: "No one can practice acupuncture anymore!" There are no statistics. We do not know how correct his statement is. It is a fact that the *Great Encyclopedia of Needling and Burning (Zhenjiu dacheng)* by Yang Jizhou (1522–1620) appeared in 1601. An extensive, impressive work, published a mere three years after Li Shizhen's encyclopedia of pharmaceutics. So the literary zeniths of acupuncture and pharmaceutics lie close together. Yet, they are so far from each other. Pharmaceutics had been steadily developing since antiquity. Li Shizhen's encyclopedia remains the definitive work. It has been reprinted many times—there are at least fifty-six editions from imperial times up to the present. As for new publications, in the seventeenth, eighteenth, and nineteenth centuries, small, manageable pharmaceutics books for the practitioner became available.

For acupuncture, things looked different. Regardless of the publication of the *Great Encyclopedia of Needling and Burning* in the year 1601— which was reprinted at least fifty-three times before 1911—two decades after the initial publication, another renowned physician and author, Zhang Jiebin (ca. 1563–1640), declared that there were no more experts in acupuncture! Again, there are no statistics. Was Zhang Jiebin an opponent of acupuncture who overlooked the facts? Or was he describing the facts? It is hard to say. The state of affairs a century later is clearer. Again, a renowned physician and author on acupuncture, Xu Dachun, expressed himself. We read about Xu in the previous chapter and are familiar with his basic views. He openly stated: "Acupuncture can provide wonderful healing!" His statement is a complaint about reality. He had no reason to exaggerate. He wrote that acupuncture had fallen into disregard and was no longer frequently practiced. In antiquity, the procedure was highly treasured; in his time, no one mentioned it anymore. That was in 1754.

This is beyond astonishing. Most Westerners today consider acupuncture to be a core aspect of Chinese medicine—though this is historically not entirely correct. Acupuncture was, in antiquity and for a thousand years up to the twelfth or thirteenth century, the only therapeutic procedure in Chinese medicine. Pharmaceutics remained a nonmedical therapeutics, free of theory. Beginning in the twelfth or thirteenth century, pharmacy was included in medical therapeutics—and competed with acupuncture. Under the Ming and Qing, the Song teachings ossified to mere formalities and pharmaceutics was not harmed at all. It managed quite well without pharmacological interpretation. Whoever wanted to could think and act pharmacologically. There were plenty of instructions, for example in Li Shizhen's *Encyclopedia* of 1598. But theories were not needed. Regardless of the plausibility of the theories or political necessity, whoever wanted to could depend solely on the effects of individual drugs and prescriptions—without the "empty theoretical drivel of the Song era" that Xu Dachun hated so much.

But acupuncture—it was inseparably linked to these theories. It flourished in antiquity, but was now fading away. Dwindling interest in the teachings of systematic correspondences of all things could, from our perspective, be closely connected with a declining interest in Confucian teachings. Xu Dachun named two other reasons for the diminishing attraction of acupuncture: First, the needle procedure is more difficult to learn than pharmaceutics. It is not easy to remember the exact locations of the insertion points, and the techniques—filling up, draining, and so on—are complicated. And, of course, there are different sorts of needles. All forgotten. Second, people didn't like being stuck with needles anymore. Acupuncture is bloodletting, too, and people could no longer stand the sight of blood. Taking pharmaceutics is much less problematical.

A careful reading of the remarks of Xu Dachun reveals that he did not merely uncover the pharmaceutics of "empty philosophizing." He also transformed acupuncture into a mechanical technique. The contents of the yin-yang and the five agents doctrines were suspect to him. He avoided these as much as possible. In his view, the only right way to proceed was consistent rejection of the Song-era theories in pharmaceutics, followed by detheorization of the needle therapy. Pharmaceutics could live with that. This we have seen. But acupuncture? How stable was and is its effect without the instructions of theory? It is hard to say—even today.

Since the 1970s, experiments have been conducted in many places to replace the ancient Chinese theories of systematic correspondences with modern scientific interpretations. This is a difficult venture and, until now, has failed to produce any noteworthy outcome. But in Xu Dachun's time? At that point, the old theory had faded and there was no new one in sight! Can acupuncture survive without the plausibility of its ancient theories? Are its effects real enough to be convincing beyond the plausibility lent to them by Confucian social theory? In the Qing dynasty, these questions were answered with a clear "No!" Acupuncture did not survive. A bit of routine here and there. Folk medicine adopted much of this. What has been thought up and introduced in the past is continued in folk knowledge and folk tradition. That is a good thing. But for intellectuals? Acupuncture had died. Or as Xu Dachun put it: It had been forgotten!

In the seventeenth and eighteenth centuries, another development began that was detrimental to acupuncture: the entrance of barbers into therapeutics. This is not at all foreign to us. For centuries in Europe, in some places in Germany up to the middle of the twentieth century, barbers maintained a steady position in the spectrum of healers. In China in the Qing era, haircutters were indispensable, because fashion required men to shave from the forehead to the middle of the head. Haircutters then also began to offer massages to their clients. The so-called push and pull massage, *tuina,* soon became popular.

Only a few books were written on this procedure. But countless manuscripts are available. They transmitted this knowledge beneath the conventional level of scholarship. What were its advantages? Tuina massage was cheap, safe, and without side effects. It could achieve effects similar to pharmaceutics: a clever tuina masseur could trigger sweating, vomiting, or laxative effects in patients through his manipulations, which saved expensive medical costs.

The masseurs applied pressure to the same points where acupuncturists stuck their needles, and could even treat children without risk—a clientele that was out of reach for the needle therapists. Treatments by acupuncturists were expensive, and needles were thick, painful and their application not without dangers. Even the emperor himself was treated with tuina massage. His masseurs were especially clever. During the massage, they kept two fingers free on each hand. With these, they produced clicking noises that sounded like birds chirping. The mightiest rulers would soon fall into a soft sleep. Imperial success flung open the door for the new therapy, and acupuncture lost a large portion of its clientele. How convincing and indispensable could the needle effects have been if they were thus forced into the background by massage? In 1822, the authorities condemned and banned further application of acupuncture as unsafe. There were hardly any trustworthy experts left.

62 | No Scientific Revolution in Medicine

The centuries following the decline of the Song dynasty to the end of the empire in 1912 were a time of searching. There is no question that the old explanatory models possessed a certain dynamic of their own. But fundamentally new things? There were a couple of initiatives, but no one author was able to provide a blueprint to give medicine truly new momentum. There had been such new momentum in the Han era. After the innovation was expressed and accepted, routine followed. And there was new momentum again in the Song era. Once the innovation had been expressed and accepted, routine ensued here, too.

Thomas Kuhn (1922–1996) drew a lot of attention with his thesis on "scientific revolutions." He called the explanatory models of science "paradigms." A paradigm, he explained, comes to dominance by a revolution. While it is dominant, all explanations of the relevant scientific discipline are taken from this paradigm. This is called the phase of "normal science." Eventually, it becomes evident that the paradigm cannot solve all questions. Contradictions increasingly pile up. Sometimes these contradictions are so flagrant that a revolution brings a new paradigm to dominance, and the phase of "normal science" begins anew under the new explanation model.

There has never been a revolution in this sense at any time in the history of medicine. In therapeutics overall, and in medicine in particular, new momentum never came from within. The new impetus was also never stimulated by contradictions between the plausibility of an explanatory model and the reality of the physical organism. The logic of plausibility is not measured by the reality of the bodily organism. Thus, no contradiction could build up and stimulate a rethinking, at least not on the most fundamental level. A new dynamic only arises if something fundamental changes that is external to medicine.

There have always been movements. The movements in the Mongolian, Ming, and Qing eras were certainly noticeable and perhaps even traumatic for the contemporaries. But they were not fundamental. They could not fundamentally question the structures of the imperial period. The Neo-Confucianism of the Song era was elevated by the Qing dynasty to official state doctrine—as hollow and shallow as this doctrine was for most scholars. Within these real and ideal structures, thoughtful people sought orientation and looked around. They remained prisoners. In culture, as in medicine, there is no special new path, and no special escape. First, a real or ideal way out must be shown by the overriding structures. The end of the imperial era let this new path emerge.

63 | The Discovery of New Worlds

We interrupted our look at Europe at the time when Vesalius so impressively demonstrated the reality of human anatomy with the help of his illustrator, Titian's student Jan Steven van Kalkar, a contemporary of the sixteenth century. We must also mention Leonardo da Vinci (1452–1519). Half a century before van Kalkar's drawings, da Vinci offered previously unknown views into the reality of the interior of the body. The dramatic transition from the hitherto conventional two-dimensional presentation method to the new plasticity can hardly be imagined. Da Vinci was a painter, architect, technician, and observer of nature. But he was not a physician. He did not publish his anatomical studies. From 1570 until late in the eighteenth century, they fell into obscurity and were forgotten. Had van Kalkar known about them? Possibly. Vesalius may have learned from da Vinci. In any case, Vesalius and Jan Steven van Kalkar's drawings pulled back the curtain further than any physician before: The stage is open! Look at all there is in the body! The audience did not have to be asked twice.

There was so much to see there. So much to compare: What is normal? What is healthy? What is sick? Can it be measured? In Italy, a new monetary economy developed. Wealth, prosperity, and power no longer depended on feudal or Church privileges. The citizen as tradesman could amass countable, measurable forms of wealth, of prosperity—and he did! Health or illness—that is linked to prosperity. Was this why weighing, comparing, measuring, and counting found such early entrance into medicine in Europe? Possibly, but not necessarily. Wealth, prosperity, and power were also linked very closely with countable, measurable coins in China. However, that did not affect the view of the body there.

More important, however, was the incentive to discover new worlds. Hadn't Columbus stepped onto a new stage shortly before Vesalius lifted the curtain? That was the first New World. Others soon followed. There was so much to see. The Americas, Africa, Asia. Not everyone could board one of the small, swaying ships. Not everyone could go to distant places. But there were alternatives. Everyone wanted to be an explorer, but not everyone wanted to risk the dangers of the high seas. In that case, the dissecting table was preferred. There was so much to discover there. It was a bloody affair, and adventurous, too. After all, it was not that easy to get a corpse. Vesalius had to have his eyes and ears everywhere. Did the priest's secret mistress recently die at his private residence? Get there quickly, steal her in the monk's absence, skin her quickly to make her unrecognizable, and off to work. This was surely as exciting as confronting a native from another land.

And fame could be attained by the explorer's travels in the body's interior! Columbus became famous for discovering America. We have already discussed Vesalius. His contemporary Gabriele Fallopio (d. 1562) became famous for his discovery of the fallopian tubes. Giovanni Battista Canano (d. 1579) and Girolamo Fabrizio ab Aquadependente (d. 1619) became famous for discovering and describing the vein valves. Morgagni (1682–1771) became famous for showing more clearly than others that the organs were the site of disease. Marie François Xavier Bichat (1771–1802) became famous for researching and discovering the tissues as the site of disease. And Karl von Rokitansky (1804–1878) also became famous! Not for discovering important anatomical details. That was not his goal at all. He was not an anatomist, but a pathologist. It was the sheer number of his trips into the "new world" that gained him eternal renown: he applied the knife and entered the body's interior, well known to him, many thousands of times. He saw a lot on these trips, interpreted, explained, and got caught up in speculations at the end of his career, but his early fame did not fade.

The anatomists' and pathologists' voyages of exploration into the body's interior brought much reality to light. For medicine, this reality was not yet meaningful. What does it mean if a physician knows about the vein valves or sees fallopian tubes? Very little. Medicine is interested in answering: What is normal? What is sick? Why does the normal turn into sickness? How can sickness be returned to normality? This is where interpretation begins. This is the start of uncertain terrain, based on plausibility and reality. Observers explored the terrain of interpretation for four or five centuries. Piece by piece, reality was wrested from this ground. Piece by piece, it was illuminated by plausibility.

64 | Paracelsus: A Tumultuous Mind with an Overview

Many felt and many were aware that Galen's antiques did not belong in the new era. They made every effort to build a new edifice of knowledge. But where did the blueprint come from? Where did the building blocks come from? Many confusing model images offered plausibility. How could all of this be brought together? China, as we have seen, was still caught in a cage, with bars as solid then as they had ever been, made of the worldview of correspondences. In this cage, Chinese observers of nature strayed from corner to corner and could not escape. In Europe, observers of nature were likewise lost, but on a much vaster terrain. They tried to find safety in a new cage.

Many master builders set up models and hoped that people would soon crowd in. They were often disappointed. The bars were too weak; the holes in the grating too obvious. A large number could never be taken prisoner. When people did crowd in, it was only for a short time. And yet, later master builders learned from their predecessors; they made efforts to suggest a more stable cage. We have already mentioned

Hildegard von Bingen (1098–1179). She was one of the early European master builders. Her cage still exists today. A millennium after the abbess set up her lattice bars, some people still feel comfortable in it at the beginning of the twenty-first century. Although there are other roomier cages, people come to hers of their own free will. Paracelsus (1493–1541), a contemporary of Vesalius, is the next master builder we will look at more closely.

Paracelsus was exceedingly controversial even during his own lifetime. He was a master builder of a cage of ideas that no one could tolerate for long. And yet it was influential, puzzling, and has been hotly debated to the present day. For us, one sentence of the many that Paracelsus wrote stands out: "There is nothing inside the body that is not observable from the outside."[52] The gist of this, roughly translated, is that for Paracelsus, the plausibility of the outside of the human body was sufficient to interpret the processes inside of the body. This is the antithesis of Vesalius's position. Unfortunately, most of Paracelsus's biographical details are uncertain. But it is possible that, as a young man in Villach, in the province of Carinthia, he came into contact with metalworking at the foundries close to the ore mines. He didn't yet know anything of Hippocrates and Galen. He later cut the ancient greats down to size and trusted solely in his own experiences. Was this attributable to his view of the metal works in the vicinity of the Carinthian ore production? It is imaginable that it was here that he had the impulse and saw the model image for his view of the organism: a simmering, hissing, occasionally malodorous vessel, in which the sulfuric, salt-like, and mercurial are unified.

This is not modern chemistry by a long shot. It is also not real alchemy. But it is the transference of observed regularities in nature onto the assumed regularities in the organism. Paracelsus, in contrast to Vesalius, did not look into the body—and yet he saw what happens there. Not that he had already found the words that convince us today. But that is not the point at all. The important thing is that he compared the processes in the body with the processes he had seen at the metal foundry in Carinthia, or somewhere else.

He had observed that in nature, external to humans, there are flammable substances. There is an underlying principle to these substances. This he called sulfur, the principle of the sulfuric, that which is oily and flammable. Then there is what remains in nature after something is burned, the ashes. This is the principle of salt, the earthlike, the remains. It withstands even the power of fire. And there is yet a third thing in nature: the principle of the fluid, the moveable, the mercurial. With this term, he referred to everything that vaporizes, flows, precipitates in sublimates. Paracelsus knew no chemical elements. He recognized principles of effect. That was the beginning. Later, elements emerged in place of these principles of effect. That was the real breakthrough. But Paracelsus was close to it.

Fire possessed the greatest meaning for him. It was the most important power that Paracelsus recognized to dissociate, to separate. Above all was the cinder from the agent. Again, what influence was exerted by the ore production in Carinthia? In many natural substances, there is an arcanum: a hidden active substance. This had to be dissolved out, separated from the cinders and poison. The agent can be a transparent, volatile gas—and yet be as powerful as a heavenly body. The agent hides in plants. Whoever distills them can overcome the *seeds* of every illness. Don't believe any of that nonsense of the four humors doctrine! Paracelsus was a man of clear words. He tried out many substances as the carriers of hidden agents: copper sulfate, antimony chloride, arsenic and bismuth compounds, and others. Bars in a cage that many others wanted to hold onto.

But Paracelsus used a broad variety of building blocks. The tumultuous mind, as Lichtenthaeler called him,[53] had a broad overview. He believed illnesses could be attributed to five causes: the influence of the stars, the effects of poisons, the effects of natural disposition, the effects of the spirit, and the effects of God. That does not sound so distant from us at all. Many might declare themselves in agreement with this panorama, even today. Paracelsus was a physician, but he did not create a medicine. His therapeutics encompassed science and the numinous. The lattice of his cage proved to vary in its strength. Theology, magic, philosophy, and alchemy. Great, wonderfully beautiful, narrow and winding architecture.

And yet, as master builder, Paracelsus was doomed to fail from the start. He linked the reality of the metallurgic melting kitchens in Carinthia with the belief in God. That is absolutely sensible. But such a cage could no longer be built, even in the sixteenth century. Each potential inhabitant found some fault or other in the plans. In addition, Paracelsus was no master of marketing. Charismatic, yes. But he was also a fanatic who made a big mistake. He clothed the new things that he believed he saw in a new terminology that only he could understand. But the secret of the art of persuasion to the new consists in delivering new things in familiar words. Then it does not seem quite so offensive.

65 | Durable and Fragile Cage Bars

Didn't we say the master builders learned from each other? Paracelsus, the outcast who was reviled, miserable, and died in poverty, had a student who was a Flemish nobleman: Johann Baptist van Helmont (1579–1644). Van Helmont was the first to use the word *gas;* his teacher Paracelsus had still called what is volatile "chaos." Van Helmont not only coined the term, he was also the first to clearly define it: "Matter bodies have a spirit in themselves and at times change totally into this spirit. It is not that it truly resides in the body. . . . It has 'condensed' itself into a matter body."[54] Van Helmont did experiments to find out more about this spirit that he called gas. He identified carbon dioxide, sulfur dioxide, and chlorine gas. That sounds good. But the context must be considered. It doesn't sound quite as good today. He believed he saw five kinds of gas: wind gas, fat gas, dry gas, soot gas, and forest gas. These were pure products of thought, with weak plausibility that did not convince many.

Illness exists in the organism as an inborn image, *idea morbosa.* A harmful agent must come to it and transform this image into the reality of illness. A *parasite* develops in the body that weakens the life spirit, *archaeus.* The life spirit, itself a gas, can then no longer lend health to the body. Also a nicely thought out edifice—but with a short lifespan! Yet in spite of all these fantasies, van Helmont was an observer. He helped build the new cage of European interpretation. But the cage was not standing yet. He added a few bars himself, for people to hold onto. Most of them soon broke off, but a couple proved to be durable. In therapy, he consistently followed the path of Paracelsus, who is still credited with the discovery of "medical chemistry." Van Helmont was convinced of the necessity of chemical medications and is considered the founder of "chemical therapy." At the same time, he believed in magic and the widespread idea that treating weapons with an ointment heals the wounds they have inflicted.[55]

Van Helmont and the many other builders of his time surely believed that they possessed an ordered worldview. Every element had its place: the godly, the spiritual, magical, chemical, carefully observed illnesses, and the increasing knowledge of morphology. This was certainly an orderly worldview. But it was unsuitable as a blueprint for the new cage of a new medicine. The individual parts did not fit together. What were magic and prayer really able to do? Was this the origin of the later science that could make airplanes fly and build bridges that spanned kilometers? Absolutely not. What could giving chemical substances to the organism really achieve? Was this the origin of the later medicine that learned to chemotherapeutically influence the organism? Possibly. What van Helmont and his contemporaries did not yet know was that a cage is only durable if its lattice bars are all equally durable. This was the task that lay before them. They knew nothing of it. Yet everything was directed toward the gradual removal of building blocks whose durability was doubtful and unreliable. Building machines that could fly and bridges that spanned kilometers—this was the standard!

There was still a long way to go. Who could see the signposts? Martin Luther or the Catholic Pope? The constitutional monarchy, the absolutistic central state, or small principalities? Everything existed alongside the others. And then there was news from the new worlds! Indians, Africans, and Asians stepped onto the stage! Muslims and Jews had long been around. New illnesses, epidemics, plagues, and syphilis. It was an exciting time, a time of absolute breakthrough. But where did it lead? At first, there was only one thing to do: just keep building!

66 | The Most Beautiful Antiques and the Most Modern Images in One Room

We have rushed ahead. Let us go back again to someone whom we will eternally remember as a master builder: Jean Fernel (1497–1558), a contemporary of Vesalius and Paracelsus. He created the most beautiful cage. He offered the most enticing architecture. He made use of many components that the era offered him. Above all, however, he had a tremendous model image for his plans. The title of his text: *Universa Medicina!* He was the most demanding master builder of his time. He did not create a medicine, despite the title. But he did create a comprehensive therapeutics that might have continued to exist if his era—the model image for his plans—had survived. But this was not to be. New, confusing impressions appeared at breakneck speed. As soon as a model image seemed to consolidate, it dispersed again. Ah, the distant, lovely polis democracy. How clearly it was arranged. Such harmony! Nothing was left of that era. Yet Fernel made another attempt. He was compelled to take a risk in order to make a breakthrough.

His plan of the organism was marked by hierarchy. How did he get that idea? The body itself could not have divulged it to him. Its power of expression in the sixteenth century was just as insufficient as it had been two millennia earlier. The reality was vein valves, fallopian tubes, and a few clarified details. But interpretation was not much helped by this. What is life? Who directs the processes in the organism? The questions were demanding. The answers likewise. Nicely thought out, Monsieur Fernel. You are guaranteed an honorary spot in the temple of intellectual history. But medicine? No, that was not your terrain. We understand how you convinced practicing Christians that the body was guided by a trinity of functions of the soul. You were sure of that! The body did not divulge it to you. The plausibility came from your faith.

What do the three functions of the soul rule over? The first is brain and nerves. The second is heart and arteries. The third is liver and veins. Who whispered that to you? We don't know, and you can no longer tell us. Brain and nerves, heart and arteries, liver and veins—that is reality. You have contributed an interpretation to it. Well done, but meaningless even in the mid-term. Your idea edifice was a "complicated series of steps," extending "from the rational, immortal soul right down to the organs, humors and elements, just as the hierarchy of the medieval cosmos mirrored godly and angelic powers."[56] You really did think things through to the last detail and considered how everything would have to be!

Let us examine a small excerpt of your teachings:

> Out of food, the liver produces *spiritus naturales* that spread via the venous system and provide nourishment to the vegetative functions. The finer *spiritus vitales* develop from blood and breath in the left side of the heart and spread central warmth and vitality via the body's arterial system. In the brain, the even finer *spiritus animales* are formed; they fill up the brain ventricles and flow from there through the nerves, generally thought of as pipes since Galen's time, and then to the sensory organs and muscles to effect sensation and movement. Whether in fluid or solid, *spiritus* fill the cavities of the body; as *vinculum animae*, they transfer the tasks of the *facultates* to its elementary basic parts, so that these are subjected to the thus organized whole.[57]

And those are only a few lines of your great work! Monsieur Fernel, you are credited with the culmination of Galenism. To express this a bit differently: you gave a perfect example of mannerism. You put the nicest antiques and the most modern pictures in one room. Your cage was beautifully furnished. But most of the cage bars had broken off before people had let themselves be imprisoned for even a few decades.

67 | Harvey and the Magna Carta

Someone who was actively involved in the rapid destruction of Fernel's cage was William Harvey: "Living movement is no longer subjected to a central dirigisme (be it of the soul or of the brain), but rather, it is the expression of far-reaching autonomy and interconnected action of the organic tissues that can move themselves: the muscles are, like the heart, 'just as independent life forms,' whose activity is merely modulated and coordinated by the brain and nerves." Thus wrote William

Harvey (1578–1657) in his book *On the Place Movement of Animals (De Motu Locali Animalium)*.[58] Who was Harvey? And how did he come up with such ideas?

William Harvey had read just about everything that seemed worth reading at the time, all they way back to Aristotle (including Galen, of course). He worked as an anatomist, did animal experiments, and was interested in life in the embryonic state. Harvey asked many questions about nature and the organism. And the organism answered. It told Harvey what he wanted to hear. From Aristotle, he learned about circulation as the ideal form of movement. Then there was also the path of water: from vapors to clouds, clouds to rain, and back to the earth. An eternal, usually beneficial cycle. Harvey also knew about alchemists and their distillations. He knew about the dominant role of the heart in the organism. Here, too, he concurred with Aristotle. If one had had a link to China: there too the heart had been considered the most important organ since the first century.

From Vesalius, Harvey knew that the septum of the heart is impermeable, and he had learned that there is a lung circulation from Michael Serveto and Realdo Colombo. His teacher Fabricius of Aquadependente, as we have already learned, discovered the vein valves. He knew that warmth sets things into movement, while cold leads to rigidity and solidification. He knew a lot more than this, too. But why did he have to contradict the earlier authorities? How arrogant he was to reject the central dirigisme of the soul as foundation for living movement, to regard the muscles and the heart even as "so to speak, own life forms," "whose activity is only modulated and coordinated by brain and nerves"! Harvey searched for the principles behind the visible reality and found what he already knew to be the case. It is no coincidence that he lived in England.

Has anyone examined William Harvey's political views? Did he ever mention his idea of the state, of society? Let us risk a hypothesis here, whose validity can only be speculated until someone uncovers Harvey's idea of the state and of society. For his picture of the body, of the organism, we suspect that Harvey had a model image. Perhaps he was not at all conscious of it himself, because he lived in this model image. It was the Magna Carta. Harvey transferred, intentionally or not, the Magna Carta from English constitutional reality onto the constitution of the human organism. The clergy and nobility forced the Magna Carta on the king on June 15, 1215. The final version was sealed by Henry III ten years later. It secured the freedom and rights of the landed nobility against interventions by the crown. It also intervened in trade and laid down a unified standard for masses and weights. This was almost four centuries before Harvey!

Shall we take a glance back at China at this point? Let us recall that circulation was discovered there 1,700 years before William Harvey's ideas on circulation. Granted, China's circulation was not the circulation of William Harvey. But it was an unremitting flow through two separate pipe systems. And what did we suspect as we got to know this unremitting flow? That there was a model image. The model image was the unified empire of China. Unification was not achieved by the exercise of the emperor's rule over the once independent and now unified parts. That was not yet unity.

True unity was reached when the ruler standardized measures and weights and thus set trade and mobility on their course. And so we return to England to find the physician and anatomist William Harvey, the first to see the body's real circulation. He does not merely see it. He even proves it—more than three centuries after the Magna Carta had changed constitutional reality and standardized the weights and measures of economic reality. Harvey's evidence is so straightforward that it is still used today. Plausibility and reality were wed. And it does not look as if divorce is likely.

With William Harvey, a lot of impulses and knowledge came together. But the decisive thing was his model image. It had had more than three centuries to ripen. England had constitutional continuity unlike any other place in Europe. England was the only state in Europe where erudition and stability of the political system had accompanied each other for centuries. And yet: A single scholar created the synthesis of all that knowledge, the impulses, the model image. Why not more? Why did only a single man come up with the idea of uniting the thoughts of Aristotle, the idea of the circulation, the knowledge of distillation, as well as the knowledge of the vein valves, lung circulation, and the impermeability of the septum of the heart? This will remain a great puzzle. At the beginning, we asked: Why at this place and why at this time? The question needs to be extended: Why this person? It is puzzling indeed.

Thomas Fuchs comments on this: "Instead of Galen's multipolar and decentralized physiology, Harvey suggests the principle of the heart, the sun of the microcosm. Instead of the local, there is central flow regulation: the speed and amount of the circulating blood varies depending on internal and external influences on the heart. The periphery only receives blood, is filled with it. Also, a primarily cardially conditioned pathology suggests itself: Affects influence pulses, warmth and constitution of the heart and can cause terminal illnesses by weakening the central source of warmth and nutrition."[59] Nothing else could be expected. Although we know nothing about Harvey's political views from other sources, from direct witnesses, we can risk making another hypothesis. Irrespective of the Magna Carta, Harvey, it is certain, was a loyal follower of the crown. During the civil wars, he sided with King Charles I (1600–1649), who was, as is known, prone to absolutism. That may have influenced William Harvey. The ruler is the sun in the state, the heart the sun in the organism. The heart, or rather the ruler, determines trade and mobility. If the ruler is doing well, then everything runs smoothly. If the ruler falls victim to bad influences, the state apparatus falls into ruin. This or something similar may have been William Harvey's political model image. We can see only the view of the body that he developed.

William Harvey was not a master builder of a new, comprehensive edifice of ideas. But we can call him an engineer. He focused on a problem's specific part: the circulation and the movement of the heart. On this, he wrote an important work: *De motu cordis*. And he did not mention the soul even a single time![60] And this was only a few decades after Jean Fernel's *Universa Medicina*. All that reading, and the many ideas that were included in building master Fernel's edifice of ideas! A cage that had its main and fundamental bars broken off so soon by an English engineer. Fernel and his cage are known only to a few historians today. How could such a great ideational product be lost so soon?

Harvey did not need a central soul to guide things and certainly not a trinity. His model image was the English king as *primus inter pares*—the heart as *primus inter pares.* The organs in the periphery—even the blood and the muscles—each possessed their own power to move themselves and to react to stimuli, like the clergy and the landed nobility. All used the same standardized weights and measures so that trade and change could function—circulation. But this was a different circulation than in China. Harvey was, after all, a contemporary of Francis Bacon (1561–16126), who had demanded "unadulterated experience" as the antidote to "speculation." Harvey was a speculator, but he was also an engineer. And he came from a merchant family. His father and his brothers were all merchants. Trade and change were the focus of discussion in the Harvey family. Only William took a different route and became a physician—yet he always stayed connected to the sober world of numbers, masses, and weights. He measured, calculated, and put his speculations together with the results of his calculations. He had barely published his results when someone else came along and broke everything apart again: Descartes.

68 | A Cartesian Case for Circulation

Descartes (1596–1650) may have heard of the Magna Carta. But did it make an impression on him? Probably not. He lived in France, a totally different world that had just gone through a very difficult time. Descartes' parents would have told him about the Huguenots who, supported by England, led the opposition of the estates against the monarchy. The Catholics were led by the dukes of Guise, supported by Spain. The religious wars in the country lasted until Descartes' own time. Henry IV made a change with the treaty of 1598, and the badly fragmented country recovered. From 1624 to 1642, Richelieu secured the absolute power of the crown. The humiliation of France was over. The new strength could also be recognized from the outside. Can we blame Descartes for being an unconditional centralist who could imagine a healthy, strong organism only as one ruled by a central power? Who viewed the ideal constitution of the state organism as one in which a central ruler makes decisions and all parts automatically follow? The picture he created of the organism of the human body suggests this hypothesis.

Once again, Thomas Fuchs, now on Descartes: "Instead of inherent principles, absolute laws that constitute one world of purely mechanical relationships rule over the living and the dead. The consequences of the machine paradigm are the fundamental features of automaticity of organ function, decline of self-movement and its replacement by the reflex."[61] Descartes was a more successful engineer than Harvey. Harvey had presented his discovery to his contemporaries in the handsome case of his speculations. Descartes was cruel. He took the discovery out of the handsome case and put it in a new case, one that immediately seemed more attractive. Even in England, where it could still be expected that everyone would have admired Harvey's case, with its label of Magna Carta Vitae Humanae. A bitter thing for Harvey. The label was invisible. The autonomy of the regions was obviously not as strongly anchored in people's minds as he had thought. Automation, reflex of the dependents without rights of their own, was the model that came from France and met with widespread appeal.

> These fundamental principles are realized in Descartes' idea of physiology, above all through the conceptual reinterpretations of the "life warmth" in a physical/chemical reaction process and the "life spirits" in a neuronal flow of particles. This explains, at a purely physical level, the propulsion of the body machine on the one hand and its steering and movement on the other hand. Yet, the decisive linking of propulsion and steering is achieved by circulation—now conceptualized as a mechanical "transmission belt," but also as a feedback-controlled circuit system. At the end stands, instead of Harvey's vital automaticity of the organs, their total subordination to the central nervous system.[62]

As we saw, the new packaging of Harvey's discovery by his colleague Descartes was broadly accepted. But there was also some fault-finding. No one questioned the reality of Harvey's discovery. But the case, the package! This is not very surprising. Packaging is a matter of taste. Taste is governed by aesthetics, determined less by the object that is to be packaged than by the zeitgeist and fashion. And so it was with the packaging of Harvey's discovery. Descartes was the first to make a new case. Many others followed. Let us look at a single example here.

69 | Long Live the Periphery!

Following the crown's loss of authority in the wake of the French Revolution, thirty-year-old Marie Francois Xavier Bichat (1771–1802) wrote,
on the role of the heart: "Let us stop considering this organ the only
driving force ruling the movement in the large and small vessels,
that . . . causes inflammation in them and by its impulses, various skin
eruptions, secretions, exhalations, etc. . . . The entire teaching of the
mechanists rested, it is known, on the extreme range that they allowed
the heart for its movements."[63] The model image that Descartes had
seen just 150 years earlier no longer possessed any validity for Bichat.
The plausibility of the picture that Descartes had drawn was lost the
moment centralistic absolutism disappeared. Bichat thought politically
and spoke of the heart. A pity his own heart failed him so early on. But
his impulses were transmitted. They fell on fertile soil primarily in the
German lands.

Was the Germany of the late eighteenth and the early nineteenth
centuries comparable to William Harvey's England? Indeed, there were
many small kingdoms, principalities, duchies, and so on. But a king as
primus inter pares? He did not exist. Were the German lands comparable
to the France of René Descartes? Not at all. What kind of case could be
used to package the undeniable reality of blood circulation? Bichat gave
them the key word. The hothead announced that there was absolutely
no reason to attribute a central role to the heart as Descartes had done.
Vive la périphérie! The German patriots instantly agreed. The entire
nineteenth century echoed with their praises of the periphery. Johann
Christian Reil (1759–1813), Ignaz Doellinger (1770–1841), Lorenz Oken
(1779–1851), Johann Heinrich Oesterreicher (1805–1843), Carl Gustav Carus
(1779–1868), and finally Carl Heinrich Schultz (1798–1871). Once his fel-
low German masterminds had increasingly relativized the power of the
heart, Schultz went the whole way: the "peripheral system" is responsible
for the entire circulation. This is where the blood is pulled up and sent
back to the heart. Of course! Whoever believes he could set up a central
government in Berlin to rule the periphery, listen up: The power over
the flow of the goods lies in the periphery! The capital is dependent on
deliveries! In the end, the capital was created by the periphery. Oken had

already recognized that the heart's ability to beat is because the periphery sends blood to it, and not the reverse![64]

Carl Heinrich Schultz died in 1871. That same year, a German Empire was declared, with its center in Berlin. Hardly anyone, aside from a few historians, remembered Schultz and his peripheral masterminds anymore. If only Schultz and the others had put their thoughts into writing political manifestos instead of focusing on physiological treatises! Bismarck never read physiological treatises. He even wanted to duel the pathologist Rudolf Virchow.

The Berlin Empire did not last long. It ended in 1918, in a moderate catastrophe. The unsuitable idea was adopted again, under another bad omen. That led to the ultimate catastrophe. Now, a Berlin center is at work for the third time—luckily as a republic. We will see who will be delivering to whom: the heart to the organs, or the periphery to the center. Perhaps the federalists should erect a monument to the peripherist Carl Heinrich Schultz. This time with a clear text to remember his point, which comes too late for Berlin. It is itself now at the periphery—of Europe.

70 | Out of the Waiting Shelter, into the Jail Cell

Blood circulation is reality. The interpretations of Harvey, Descartes, and the German thinkers survived on plausibility. Their ideas of the real or ideal order differed. It was inevitable that the different model images led to different pictures. Gradually, peace and order came to Europe. The systems of order came to resemble each other. And yet, no edifice of ideas had appeared that could convince many. Waiting shelters originated where the public paused for a short time, looked around, and then just traveled on with the next train.

Professor Dr. Friedrich Hoffmann (1660–1742) designed one of these waiting shelters. His "Hoffman's drops" are still familiar to some older pharmacists, even today. He gained early renown as a physician. The Prussian kings Frederick I and Frederick William I liked the drops and promoted him to be their personal physician. Hoffmann was not only an architect; he was also a property developer. This made him a worthy colleague of Dr. Jean Fernel. But the model image was already a very different one: technology! The goddess of a new era. It was also present in the human organism. This personal physician saw the organism as a machine with inherent hydraulics. A nerve fluid pulsates that arises from the ether that enters the body with the breath and is driven in the body by the contraction and expansion of fibers.

"The most important movement is, according to Hoffmann, the constant circulation of blood. It protects the body from decaying and thus provides life. Disturbances in movement are the direct cause of illness . . . above all, they change the constitution and flowing properties of the blood. Increased speed increases the friction and warmth in the body. With slowed movement, the substances separate, clump up and clog the vessels. Harmful substances are no longer filtered out and excreted, so that decay can set in, or the blood clots, overstretches the vessels and finally causes them to break open."[65] Hoffmann created a new medicine. He recognized the laws of nature as the only entry to reality. He accepted nothing else for his edifice. And yet, he remained embedded in his interpretations of reality, in plausibility from A to Z. And he had success.

This is noteworthy—the man had clinical success as a physician. He was the first professor for medicine at the newly founded university in Halle. His patients returned to health. Important people recommended him to others. Prussian kings trusted him and recovered. Whoever heals is right. Then many are right! Who could judge who is really right? Hoffmann was one of those who could welcome a crowd of visitors into his edifice of ideas for a short time. These visitors revered his writings; they studied and discussed the furnishings of his building. But they soon realized that the floors were crooked and the furniture was wobbly, and so they departed again. The books remained. Nothing else.

It was no different for John Brown (1735–1788), a Scottish physician and a slave to drink and opium. No wonder he attributed illness to two primary poles: excessive stimulation and insufficient stimulation! Health lies somewhere in between. The effects of excessive stimulation must be reduced; the effects of insufficient stimulation strengthened. Granted, most people are insufficiently stimulated. Especially in Scotland, back then. And to enhance stimulation? For that, nature has given us alcohol and opium. But also spices, rich meals, camphor, and sports. Then there are also the poor souls who are always overstimulated. They can be healed with vomiting, bloodletting, and laxatives. It was quite simple, this medicine!

Several of his wig-wearing contemporaries took John Brown seriously. Especially in Germany. Here they either knew nothing of John Brown's prison years, or it did not bother anyone. In fact, only in Germany was he really taken seriously. From the waiting shelter of Professor Friedrich Hoffmann the German thinkers moved into John Brown's jail cell—and some stayed for the rest of their lives. They included him in the teachings of the Romantic era, heralded the bipolar universe, and wrote scholarly essays about his system. They applied his theories and killed fifteen-year-old Auguste Schlegel, daughter of Caroline Schlegel. Schelling liked it. Not the death of Auguste Schlegel, but the method of treatment.[66] He was a philosopher, after all. In philosophy, plausibility removes itself from reality even more often than in medicine.

71 | Sensations That Pull into the Lower Parts of the Body

Franz Anton Mesmer (1734–1815) was a scientist; as such, he had an extreme aversion to demons and spirits. He clearly denounced exorcism and looked for healing powers in nature. In fact, nature was his only model image. He forms a trinity with John Brown, whom we are already acquainted with, and Samuel Hahnemann, whom we will get to know shortly. As different as these three contemporaries were, their therapeutics were identical in a very particular respect. Together they form an exception in the entire history of medicine. The three are united by a common attribute: they created the only idea systems in the two-thousand-year history of medicine that arose primarily out of the expressiveness of the organism. That had never happened before, and it has not happened since.

In antiquity and many times since then, in both Europe and China, we have observed that a fundamental change in the reality of life—

economic, political, social—has produced a fundamental change in the view of nature, which in turn causes a fundamental new view of the individual human organism. Out of that, a new view of sickness and health ultimately develops. And now, in the eighteenth and early nine-teenth century, there are three contrasting examples: Brown, Mesmer, and Hahnemann. All three were led not by preconceived images, but rather by very concrete experiences.

John Brown, in and out of prison, learned about the effects of alco-hol and opium (incidentally, he preferred high doses of these "medica-tions"), cold baths, and spices through his own experience, and made up his own theory based on that. Franz Anton Mesmer played around with magnets. All he knew about them was that they contained, and seemed to emit, invisible natural powers. Otherwise, how could iron filings behave so strangely without touching the magnet at all? It had to be investigated. He was a scientist, or at least he believed himself to be one, and the experiment stands at the forefront of the separation of plausibility and reality.

On July 28, 1774, the time had come. Whatever her problem was, the maid Oesterlin felt terrible: she suffered from madness, rage, vomiting, fainting spells, toothaches, and earaches. Blood rushed impetuously to her head. Franz Anton Mesmer took refuge in nature: "I brought her three artificial magnets and laid one onto her stomach and one on each foot. This quickly raised astonishing sensations inside her. She experi-enced a painful flowing of a very fine material that moved around but in the end settled in the lower parts of the body and freed her from all further attacks for the next six hours."[67]

Franz Anton Mesmer concluded that there is an "animal magnetism" and an "animal gravity." Entirely natural. No hocus pocus. The magnet can influence the organism. Mesmer continued to think about his dis-covery; by 1775 he was sharing his thoughts with his colleagues. People were impressed. Again, many wig-wearers nodded in approval and wrote scholarly papers. After all, Franz Anton Mesmer was not a former convict like John Brown; he was the dean of one of the most renowned medical faculties in Europe: Vienna.

Mesmer now traveled extensively, appearing as a magician who created wonderful effects with his magnets. A minor scandal, the ostensible curing of a blind pianist, detracted from this for only a short time. Above all it was Paris, from 1778 on, where Mesmer was in demand. The group sessions in his salon! The sensations that permeated the body and pulled "in the lower parts of the body" as with the maid Oesterlin. Everyone wanted to be there. This was convincing. As for the theory that Mesmer came up with afterward—lack of irritability of the muscles that is restored by the magnet—few were interested. His examination commission reported to his majesty: Effects yes, during but not due to the therapy. Imagined by those seeking healing.[68] Poor Mesmer. His *cage aux folles* was mercilessly torn down, just like the Bastille.

72 | Homeopathy Is Not Medicine

Samuel Hahnemann (1755–1843) was the third in the alliance. He was from a poor family and had to translate English (and later French and Italian) medical and pharmaceutical texts to finance his studies. He was one of the best-read medical students of his time and thus also one of the most-educated doctors. He did not have a high opinion of John Brown, whom he accused of having book learning without practical relevance. But there were also similarities: John Brown had his self-experiment with alcohol and opium; Samuel Hahnemann found his therapeutics in a self-experiment with cinchona bark. It was not medical therapeutics, but at least it was therapeutics—and it was very successful at that.

In the course of one of his translations, Samuel Hahnemann uncovered a clue in British author William Cullen's remark that cinchona bark was effective against malaria. The reasoning surprised Hahnemann: cinchona bark, according to Cullen, strengthens the digestive organs! Samuel Hahnemann was not convinced and he decided to experiment on himself. He did not notice any strengthening of the digestive organs. Instead, he felt like he did when he had malaria as a student. This was exciting—the discovery stimulated Samuel Hahnemann to such an extent that he thought further: perhaps here was the hidden basic principle that applies to all sickness.

Hahnemann was a man aware of his responsibility. He conducted further experiments on himself, his family, and later on his students. Always on healthy people. This was a new idea! Hahnemann's insight was that a substance shows its effect on the healthy. These effects are like a kind of illness. The more effective the substance, the stronger the pharmaceutically induced symptoms. Hahnemann observed and observed. He recorded his observations and finally came to the conclusion that medication heals the same illness in the sick that it produces in the healthy. This is particularly true for chronic illnesses. First, the chronicity is suppressed through the medical illness. Then, the influence of the medication disappears and the patient returns to health. No illness is like another.

Did Hahnemann know that Chinese doctors had had similar thoughts since the thirteenth century? Every sickness, as he and the Chinese followers of the systematic correspondences pharmacology taught, is an individual problem requiring an individual treatment. In the foreground is the exact observation of an illness. That takes time. Additionally, the illnesses caused by medications in the healthy must be carefully observed. There can be up to a thousand symptoms. That also takes time. But that is the experience that Hahnemann demands as the foundation of serious medication therapy. He does not find this seriousness in conventional therapists: he calls them "the humble great-grandchildren of myopic great-grandparents."[69]

Hahnemann was not myopic. He saw that every plant had been given its own medication principle from its creator, which could not be removed from the plant in any way—and certainly not by chemical processes. This medication principle that lives in the plant like a spirit works on the life power that resides in the body like a spirit, in the stomach. Here, the two spirits meet. If they are to have their effects, the patient must have faith. Not in the therapy, but in his physician. This, too, is cross-cultural. Two millennia before, a Chinese text stated that he who believes not in medicine but in spirits should not be treated at all, for no effect can be expected.

Hahnemann was successful with his doctrine. There were critics who could not make sense of his teachings, especially Hahnemann's idea that the strength of the medications could be increased by mixing them with alcohol in fluid tinctures or applying them as powder in lactose rubs. Yet even many critics of his theory had to conclude that giving medications in accordance with Samuel Hahnemann's instructions showed effectiveness. And so it has remained until today.

Hahnemann needed only a few bars for his cage. He proceeded without explaining how illnesses come about. With no thought to the causes of illness, no thought to prevention is needed. There was also no attempt to collect illnesses into groups. Every illness stands on its own. Where others planned extensive edifices of idea, Samuel Hahnemann remained humble. *Similia similibus*. Similar with similar. That is enough. Homeopathy is not medicine. It trusts a principle. It needs no laws of nature, and so it needs no science, either. The effect of the medication cannot be traced back to chemical laws. It is the spirit that was given individually to each substance by the creator. This is numinous therapeutics—created by a physician who was very well read and, as such, one of the most educated representatives of his discipline.

Where do plausibility and reality meet here? This is a fascinating puzzle. A self-experiment with substances on the healthy—is the result reality? What lends plausibility to Hahnemann's teachings? Is it the fear of the "strong" medicine of the allopaths that leads people to the "potentiated" weak medicine of the homeopaths? Or is it the insistence that each individual is different? Everyone must be thoroughly questioned and observed. Every illness is unique! Generalizations are unreliable. Everyone must be taken very seriously in his or her suffering.

That was different in the normal practice of medicine at that time, and it is different in the normal practice of medicine today. Normal medicine prefers to understand illnesses as mass goods, for which the pharmaceutical industry produces mass goods. Conventional medical business sees illness as a deviation from the norm and healing as reintegration into the norm. Values—liver values, blood values, lipid values—must be normal. There is no individuality, even among those who feel healthy. Sometimes a patient does not notice a deviation from the norm at all. Only the diagnosis shows a deviation from the norm. None of this is included in Hahnemann's teachings. There, illness is a subjective state and can be understood and treated only individually. The human becomes an individual through illness. This sounds good and seems plausible. Reality is not needed. No anatomy, the idea is already enough. This was a self-experiment with long-lasting consequences.

John Brown has fallen into obscurity; his cage was attractive only in the short term. The same fate awaited Franz Anton Mesmer; his *cage aux folles* also soon broke apart. Only Hahnemann's cage has lasted to the present day. That is surprising, considering how economical his architecture is. From Germany to Russia to India, inmates voluntarily crowd into Samuel Hahnemann's waiting shelter. They have settled there cozily. Many rooms were set up, though, to demarcate oneself from other visitors. The Nazis liked it a lot, and spent unprecedented amounts of money to elucidate the reality behind the plausibility via science—with no results, like all scientific research on homeopathy to date. And yet, the guests stay. They form little groups that conflict with one another, but they stay.

The search for recognition as an individual seems to unite people, or at least in places where people's individuality is not recognized socially. In the United States, it is different. There, Hahnemann's teachings unfolded their plausibility merely in the short term, as a European souvenir. Today, homeopathy's light is weak at best there. Whereas in Germany, Russia, and India, its plausibility gleams as brightly now as it did then.

This much remains: Hahnemann's doctrine is the only long-term, successful therapeutic doctrine that began with a clinical observation. The interpretation came later. Though Hahnemann was educated as a physician, his interpretation of what he observed was not medical, but numinous. This interpretation is unacceptable to many scientists. For many practitioners, it has plausibility. The effect itself is not decisive for the acceptance of the theory. Whoever accepts the interpretation because he or she finds it plausible considers successes of the therapy as proof of the correctness of the theory. Whoever rejects the interpretation as implausible dismisses the successes of the therapy as anecdotal, as random.

It is hard to see why followers find Hahnemann's interpretation plausible. Perhaps patients accept Hahnemann's teachings because of their aversion to the heroic therapies of conventional medicine. It might also lie in the guaranteed treatment as an individual. It is not quite discernible, and that is the fascinating thing about homeopathy.

73 | "God with Us" on the Belt Buckle

John Brown, Franz Anton Mesmer, and Samuel Hahnemann are marginal figures in the history of therapeutics. Let us again turn to medicine. Or better: let us turn to the countless architects and engineers who,
in retrospect, were involved in creating a new medicine. Gradually, it
became clear which blueprint became the focus of public attention. Two
authors symbolized the contradiction that still permeated Europe. On the
one hand, there was the pastor and population statistician Johann Peter
Süssmilch (1707–1767). He wrote a work on therapeutics and announced
with certainty: all illnesses come from God! On the other hand, there
was the physician and propagator of public health Johann Peter Frank
(1745–1821). He wrote a work on medicine and announced with certainty:
people get sick because social conditions make them sick.

The thoughts of J. P. Süssmilch were on their way out. The knowledge
of J. P. Frank pointed to the future. They considered the individual's
health to be the foundation of the strength of the modern state, which
depended on healthy workers for manufacturing and healthy soldiers
for the military. Johann Peter Frank and some of his contemporaries
rang in a new era. Therapeutics was adapted to the explanatory models
that guaranteed the efficient performance of the modern state. Things
were now moving toward putting planes in the air and building bridges
across straits.

The ideas of J. P. Süssmilch increasingly receded into the background—
from the seven-day week to just on Sundays. From Monday to Saturday,
other realizations dominated: productivity and fitness for military service
through science and technology. Blessings were distributed on Sundays,
and in war: "God with us" was engraved on uniform belt buckles. But
in the production of weapons, other explanation patterns promised the
desired success: physics, chemistry, and technology. These were the materials out of which the new cage bars were forged for a new medicine.
In the nineteenth century, it was finally there. The Romantic era, under
the leadership of Schelling, can be understood as the last gasp of those
who did not want to be forced into the cage of pure science and technology. Their edifice soon collapsed. The homeopaths offered a nonreligious

alternative accommodation, but remained outsiders, as they have always been for two long centuries. The pull of the new medicine continued to increase.

For the second time in history, a medicine was created that was distinct from all other forms of therapeutics. It understood the organism solely on the foundation of laws of nature, chemistry, and physics, via biochemistry and biophysics. For the decision makers in society, these are the only cage bars that have endured. They went into this cage voluntarily and took the overwhelming majority of the population with them. Here lay strength, measurably and visibly. Only a few had the courage and strength to remain outside.

74 | Medicine Independent of Theology

The enthusiasm of those years, hardly understandable today, led the British physician's journal *Lancet* to proclaim in 1850: "Medicine Independent of Theology." Everyone knew this really meant: finally. That was the mood of the decision makers. Now everything came together quickly. In the foreground, the great enlightenment stood: reliability and reproducibility of knowledge. Reliability means one can be sure that this knowledge provides many answers now, and one can be just as sure that this knowledge will provide even more answers in the future. Reproducibility means one can ask the question everywhere in the world, in every situation, and the answers are always the same. That must have been a fascinating experience. Who can imagine it today?

Never before had there been knowledge that was accepted as reliable and reproducible across religious boundaries! The knowledge of chemistry, physics, and technology began to change the living environment. It accompanied the Europeans on their expeditions out into the world and, being reliable and reproducible, assisted in subjecting foreign peoples to European rule. It was natural that the new medicine had to be built solely on this foundation. Only the new medicine was reliable and reproducible. As in Greek antiquity, a single view of the body and the functions of its organism, in healthy as in sick days, founded on natural laws, pushed itself into the foreground. No one could fail to hear the promise: the laws that make society productive and fit for war also make the individual organism healthy and fit for work.

Plausibility increasingly coincided with reality. Morphology had been researched for centuries and it had been seen ever more clearly. Now, for the first time in the history of humankind, chemistry and physics, functions and processes could be explained. Now the right questions were being asked of the body, and it offered countless answers. Its own expressive power remained as limited as it had always been. But in response to the appropriate questions, its expressiveness seems limitless. Chemistry, physics, and technology formed the grammar of the questions that were asked. The body responded to these questions and visibly revealed itself.

75 | Virchow: The Man of Death as the Interpreter of Life

A pathologist made the breakthrough. Rudolph Virchow (1821–1902), a physician who had made the assessment of death the focus of his daily routine, was the first to cross the finish line in the race to be the foremost interpreter of life! From today's perspective, we would not unconditionally agree that his explanation completely corresponds with reality. But this is a minor consideration. The important thing is that a jury of his contemporaries declared him the winner. We are only left with the question: why?

Answering this is much easier than in earlier centuries. Our thanks go to the historian Renato G. Mazzolini, who investigated the question for Virchow that we have been asking for the entire history of medicine: "To what extent can sociopolitical ideas influence the development of scientific theories?"[70] Mazzolini provides us with everything we need. He will be quoted at length here. If we stand on his shoulders, we might be able to see a bit farther.

In 1847, the "radical democrat" Julius Fröbel wrote a book entitled *A System of Social Politics*. Rudolf Virchow, then twenty-six years old, was familiar and identified with the political thought of Fröbel. Fröbel wrote:

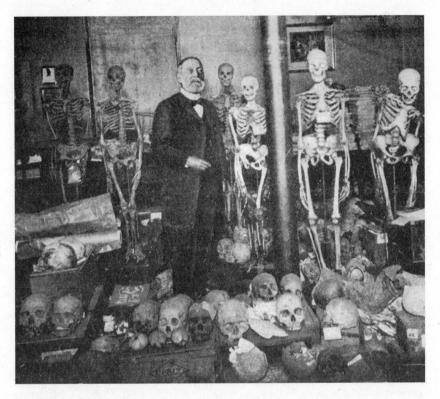

Figure 3.   Rudolf Virchow in his laboratory in the Institute of Pathology, Berlin.

"If a society exists, then it exists in the individual, of the individual and through the individual. If a community exists, then it exists for the individual, for the good of the individual." This is the crux of the message that Virchow transferred to his understanding of the organism. He regarded the body as a "facility of a social kind, where a mass of individual beings depend on each other so that every element has a special task of its own, and each element, though it may get the impetus for its task from other parts, makes the actual achievement itself." And a year later, in 1859: "What is an organism? A society of living cells, a small state, well furnished, with all accessories of higher and lower administrators, of slaves and masters, large and small."[71]

It seems it is once again time to roll out the ancient body image of Chinese acupuncture medicine. What do we see? After two millennia, not a single step of progress. Still the same old state idea, copied almost word for word from the Yellow Thearch. Yet Virchow had never heard of him; he was a child of his own time. He was struck by the ideas and impressed by model images that impacted the educated elite of central Europe in the early nineteenth century, not by Chinese model images from the first and second century BC. Is this statement—that Virchow's image of the body was based on the real or desired social structures of his time—a hypothesis like the one we have already expressed for Hippocrates and Galen, Paracelsus, Harvey, Hoffmann, and so many others? No, it is more than a mere hypothesis. This time we can thank Rudolf Virchow directly.

Not only do we know enough about Virchow's political outlook and activities outside his scientific work to know that he was a man who "maintained a keen interest in social, cultural and political questions throughout his life"; in addition, unlike earlier creators of new body images in medicine, Virchow made revealing self-observations that give us some decisive clues.

Even as a young man, Virchow considered himself to be what he termed a "whole man," elsewhere he also spoke of the "man unified in his judgment." He used this term in reference to the educated physician whose medical and political views concurred.[72] Virchow discovered this concordance in his opponents, whose statements on the biology of the body he traced back to political views that he could not share. But he also saw this concordance in himself and found it natural that his political beliefs affected his scientific ideas about the body, just as he conversely found it unavoidable to use his body image as the model for his political view of an ideal society.

But what came first? Is this the dilemma of the chicken and the egg? Not really. Virchow's political ideas determined the development of his biological theory, not the reverse. Virchow's biological theory was justified only by plausibility. He could not have derived it from the reality of the body. Neither the dead body, with which he mostly concerned himself, nor the living body offer the idea of the "organism as a society of living cells." Virchow could not prove his claim about multicelled organisms; "it was merely a hypothetical idea that stood in opposition to other theories of the structure of the so-called organized body."[73] So the great scholar is supposed to have founded his view of an ideal society on such a weak basis? This is quite unlikely, especially considering the background situation.

Mazzolini has shown decisively that Virchow brought his political convictions into medicine very early—before he did any kind of research that could have led to the development of a serious biological theory. In 1843 he finished his medical studies; in 1844 he became an assistant to Prosecutor Froriep at Berlin's Charité Hospital. In 1845, at the age of just twenty-four, he held a presentation expressing the same opinion and using the same political allegory as he did decades later. The fundamentals did not change at all. Virchow maintained his strong opinions from the outset. So this is not a question of the chicken or the egg. This man, announced with a fat banner headline in the *Chronicle of Medicine* that reads *Virchow lays the cornerstone of modern medicine*, this man—whom we thank for the first description and naming of leukemia and many other aspects of the reality of illness—this man developed his medical theories based on a predetermined political opinion, one he always kept.[74] Virchow was a master builder of his own theory of life, and he did not slowly form his building blocks over his lifetime or allow them be formed for him. He brought his own blocks from home and saw no reason at all to change them. His biological theory was not suited to exercise influence here. It was not based on a solid foundation informed by the expressiveness of the body. His biological theory was based solely on the foundation of his nonmedical convictions.

What did Virchow say right at the beginning of his career? "The new medicine takes a mechanical approach; its goal is defined as the realization of a physics of the organism. It has proven that life is merely the expression of a sum of phenomena, each occurring in accordance with the usual laws of physics. It denies the existence of an autocratic force of life and nature."[75] This claim already contains everything Virchow said in the following years about medicine and the organism. This claim is already profoundly political and allegorical.

Three main statements are unified here. Let us tackle the last one first. The newest medicine, which Virchow champions, "denies the existence of an autocratic force of life and nature." Virchow, as a republican democrat, saw no reason why a living organism should require a centrally responsible life force. A life force would mean that the organism was ruled by something he referred to as *spiritus rector*, in charge of the whole being. The individual parts comprising the whole being would have no responsibility for themselves or for the well-being of the whole, since the *spiritus rector* would determine the meaning of being and the path of development. It was just two years later that Virchow, now twenty-six years old and already a prosecutor at the Charité, elaborated on this in more detail:

> Medical ideas influenced by the dominant philosophy and political principles had developed to the extent that an integrated worldview and life philosophy was formed, of the sort that generally results when the educated physician is able to make himself into a unified man. This teleology has spread in medicine to the extent that . . . one has gotten used to considering the soul [or nerve force, life force, force of the organism, natural healing force—terms that, from our standpoint, all basically mean the same thing] to be the monarchic principle in the body.[76]

Virchow was a keen observer of his time and well educated in history. Perhaps he was an exception in his ability to connect the development of medical thought with the development of political ideas. Whatever the reason, few others adopted his view. Virchow had no use at all for the idea of the soul, the life force, or whatever else the X was called in his time. Besides, he concerned himself only with the dead. But there is more to say about this. Virchow could not see the X because only the "monarchical principle in the body" was imaginable at his time. And he rejected the monarchical principle wholeheartedly, both before he had the opportunity to conduct his own research and later. In 1847, he did not describe insights from the observation of the human body. His insights were gathered from the observation of history.

It was only in his own era that Virchow recognized change. More than others, his teacher, Theodor Schwann (1811–1882), had contributed to this change. Schwann was a man of the microscope. He used it to observe cells. To explain cell formation, he referred to crystal formation, a known process of nature. No political metaphors are found in his work. But in Schwann's writings we do find the two fundamental insights on which Virchow later founded his cellular pathology. First, animal tissues are made of cells. For this, he drew on plant cells, whose existence was already well known, as a model. Second, Schwann was the first to refer to cells in the animal organism as "individuals," following botanist Matthias Jakob Schleiden's previous description of "individual" plant cells. At the time, every elementary particle was still referred to as an individual.[77] The idea of cells as individuals fascinated Virchow. "He forever remained convinced that cells are proper individual organisms, true individuals, because they are endowed with life."[78] As individuals, these cells did not need a monarch; the power of the sovereign was transferred from the autocratic life force principle onto the individual elementary particles of the organism—on the state level as well as in the interpretation of the body: "Only in recent times, almost simultaneously with the redesign of political ideas, did a multifarious force develop alongside this unity, a force often demonstrating sovereign power; it was initially called the formation force, but soon it would be genetically ascribed to the cells themselves. Cell action, cell life, and cell force were beginning to have importance alongside the life force."[79]

Eight years later, in 1855, Virchow returned to the question of interpreting cell grouping, which could not be settled simply by observing reality. This was not about a matter of the science of reality, but rather of plausibility. What happens when a monarch loses his kingdom? Must the ship, left without a helmsman to steer its course, run aground? What can the body do if it loses its central, monarchic, autocratic life force or soul, its "life focus"? Can the body exist meaningfully at all after that? Virchow had a calming message: "Losing the unity of the living organism, through our many life foci, is not cause for alarm. Of course, we have nothing to show of unity in the sense of nerve pathology. The *spiritus rector* is missing; it is a free state of equals, albeit not equally talented individual beings, who stay together because the individuals are dependent on each other, and because certain centers of organization exist without whose integrity the individual parts could not be provided with their nutritional requirements."[80]

By now, Virchow was already thirty-four years old, the best age for scientific creativity. His statements, however, were based solely on the foundation of political allegories, as when he was twenty-four. Did Virchow lay "the cornerstone of the modern medicine" with such flimsy ideas as these? There was also something else, something that was also found in that twenty-four-year-old's presentation: "The new medicine has proved that life is merely the expression of a sum of appearances that happen to each individual in accordance with the usual laws of physics."[81] This was what made Rudolf Virchow's system of ideas so convincing. The rejection of the unfathomable, intangible X, and the radical statement that all life follows the usual laws of physics, guaranteed the practically undisputed dominance of this body image in medicine, at least for the following century.

The inclusion of all life, that is, all life processes, in the inherent laws of science, physics, and chemistry—Virchow's "usual laws of physics"— laid the cornerstone for the new medicine. No longer were nonmedical aspects of healing considered and constantly speculated about. Now, only the usual laws of physics applied; in Virchow's time, this was cell theory. He rejected what he called the "despotic or oligarchic unit" of the "humoral and solid schools" that had prevailed until then. He was skeptical of the idea that the entire body could be sick. Virchow favored the therapy of individual units, writing in 1860: "The difference is that according to the cellular view, the parts of the body comprise a societal unit and not, as in the humoral and solid schools, a despotic or oligarchic unit. It has long been recognized in successful practice that effective treatment of the sick is founded in reasoned, localized therapy, and that so-called general treatments are without success if they do not have a localized effect (sometimes unintended by the therapist)."[82]

Unity of the worldview and also unity of the world had now been achieved. The "usual laws of physics" were as valid in Berlin, Paris, and London, as they were in Tokyo and—in the future—Shanghai. The world, thus unified and on the brink of sending airplanes into the sky and building bridges over straits, was also in agreement about the innermost workings of the body. Everyone could join forces. No more pedantic nitpicking about culturally derived differences. This is what was so fascinating about the cellular pathology that the thirty-seven-year-old Rudolf Virchow had thought up in Würzburg and then presented in twenty lectures from February to April 1858 at the Pathology Institute in Berlin, lectures that were later published as a book.

Before this promising backdrop, perhaps it is unimportant that Virchow's own biological theory of life was so politically polarized and that he could lay claim to the luster of plausibility only from his political ideas. We have already looked closely at two of the basic statements in his early presentation: his opposition to the existence of a life force and monarchical and autocratic principles, and the subordination of all life processes to the usual laws of physics. One of these statements points to research and the study of reality; the other is sheer plausibility. The last of the fundamental statements (yet the first in his presentation) Virchow adhered to throughout his life is also sheer plausibility: he called the new medicine "mechanical." With this, the twenty-four-year-old stood against the "organic" viewpoint that the existence and the meaning of the separate parts of the organism could be interpreted only in terms of the existence and meaning of the whole.

Could any biological research have elicited these views in the twenty-four-year-old? From Schleiden and Schwann he had merely found out that the smallest constitutional parts in the plant and in the animal body are "individual" cells. Nothing more. Who was interested in whether they were linked "mechanically" or "organically"? Virchow was, and he knew the answer, even as a twenty-four-year old. Actually, he only expressed a political view in the cloak of biological theory. Virchow was no subscriber to the ideas of the "state organism as it was advocated at his time. . . . The term state organism comprised the idea of unity, understood as the cooperation of living parts. This was only imaginable in relation to a causality and purposefully founded whole . . . the cooperation of the parts and their relationship to the whole promoted the idea that the individual was subordinated to these, having no purpose outside the state or society."[83]

Virchow's historical knowledge led him, in an essay written in 1856, to a very clear comparison, which was aimed at sharpening his readers' consciousness of the importance of the individual:

An historian is very disposed to forget, in the abstraction of his study room, the individual living persons who comprise state and nation. He speaks of the life of nations, of national character, as if a unified power inspires and permeates all individuals, and he easily gets used to the idea of great achievements of whole nations in human historical development, without bearing in mind the many individual effects that comprise it. And yet all this action of humanity is nothing but the sum of the lives of the individual citizens. So it is also in the small state that represents the body of every plant and every animal. . . . It is self-evident that the independence of all of these parts is not absolute, but that everyone is, through his relationships, dependent on others and also they are dependent on him.[84]

Rudolf Virchow is surely the most political of all the medical thinkers we have encountered so far. He was active in Berlin's March Revolution in 1848, then banished because of his political activities from Berlin to the provincial city of Würzburg; he was in the Berlin city delegates' assembly from 1859 to his death; he was a delegate in the Prussian parliament and also later in the Reichstag.[85] He was a politician who did more than just talk: he got involved wherever his knowledge and influence could alleviate social injustice. His theory of the human organism, formulated in *Cellular Pathology,* was a theoretical edifice that, in its linking of reality and plausibility, has all the qualities of time- and person-dependent architecture.

76 | Robert Koch: Pure Science?

Virchow became the "icon of an era" because his cellular pathology made a fundamental new orientation possible. Medicine can thank him for the certainty that absolutely all questions of life can be tackled with modern scientific and technological methods. The political plausibility of this idea may have been decisive for the acceptance of cellular pathology by Virchow and other scientists. But it was not only Virchow and a few other similar antimonarchists who accepted the content and consequences of cellular pathology. All medical scientists enthusiastically embraced the new view of things, not only in Germany and Europe, but worldwide in all countries with adequate infrastructure. What was the origin of the plausibility that convinced all these people? It was the convincing power of the cumulative achievements of physics, chemistry, and technology in nonmedical areas that made it seem certain that their application to the processes in the human, animal, and plant body would answer all questions and reach medical goals.

Applying the new methods enabled Virchow and many other physicians and observers of nature to solve questions that had been demanding an answer for centuries: for example, the question of illness pathogens. Girolamo Fracastoro (1478–1553) had spoken of *seminaria*, smallest bodies, indeed even of *animalculi*, smallest animals—and no one had listened. Samuel Hahnemann had spoken of small cholera animals—and no one had listened. Even in the early nineteenth century, there was debate whether mites produced scabies or scabies produced mites. Technology, along with physics and chemistry, allowed a view into increasingly distant spaces of the all-embracing universe. The microscope, along with physics and chemistry, made it possible to view ever finer details of individual organisms. Who could doubt that the right path had at last been found?

But some things stayed the same as before. What had previously been invisible now appeared in amazing magnification. But it still did not explain itself. Interpretation was still necessary. Did mites cause scabies, or did scabies cause mites? Robert Koch (1843–1910) found convincing proof. In 1883, he discovered the pathogen of cholera and formulated the scientific postulates that have since been considered valid proof of the microbial causation of certain diseases: (1) Isolate a pathogen from a sick person. (2) Introduce the pathogen into another person. The same illness arises as in the first person. (3) Isolate the same pathogen from the second person. Pure science? Absolutely, it seemed, without a doubt!

And yet, this science is not so pure. What if Robert Koch was just lucky that his ideas were received by an era that was finally ready for them? And why was this so? Robert Koch's discovery was indisputable in most cases. Granted, the older Virchow (1821–1902) had problems with the new view of tuberculosis. But it often happens that an accomplished, celebrated older gentleman is no longer open to a new point of view—especially if it's not his own. Robert Koch prevailed with his theory of the causation of many illnesses by microbial pathogens. Right? Actually, it's exactly the opposite. Or better: yes and no. The existence of microbes is indisputable. But let us recall the Chinese model of coughing from the first century BC. It elegantly solved the observation that not everyone exposed to cold necessarily gets sick with cough. And what about microbes? Does everyone exposed to the TB pathogen in a bus or streetcar get sick? Is illness triggered solely by the amount of pathogens that find entrance into the organism? Do other cofactors exist that enable the pathogens to carry out their evil deeds? The transition from reality to plausibility began where the pathogenic theory of medicine had a monopoly.

Today, we all know what was expressed by a mere few as an all-too-weak protest more than a century ago: yes, it is evident that in many illnesses, microbes act as pathogens. But it is not right to believe that microbes as pathogens are the cause of the illness. No one listened to this protest. The pathogen was seen as the only enemy. The body is a fortress where pathogens are not allowed in. Wash your hands, keep the germs away.

77 | Wash Your Hands, Keep the Germs Away

What happened back then? Let us take a closer look. Physics and chemistry are the natural sciences. They use laws of nature to explain and understand the existence of substances, how they change, and their effects. They use laws of nature to force technology onto nature and subject it to humankind. The reaction of an acid, a base, a salt, the preparation of an organic compound out of inorganic substances, the addition of a catalyst. The generation of electricity from movement or water power. All this is reality. No plausibility is needed for this.

Against the backdrop of biochemistry, biophysics, and the use of the newest technology, plausibility then turns up after all. Why do we get sick? In the nineteenth century, some said it was because of pathogens. Others said that pathogens can invade the body only if a door has been opened beforehand. Normally, pathogens find no entrance into the healthy body. But no one listened to these voices. Pathogens had the upper hand. This is understandable. Proof of it could be grasped, or better, seen under the microscope! Today, one can hardly imagine the enthusiasm that accompanied the ascension of germ theory. The evildoer had been discovered. At last, two thousand years into the history of medicine. This was convincing—and so simple. Hygienic, sterile conditions in the operating room: what a blessing for the patient! As long as we keep pathogens at a distance, we will stay healthy. As long as we drive out the pathogens or kill them if they enter the body, we will regain health.

Perhaps Robert Koch and germ theory profited from the role models of their time. The battle had to be fought: every individual on one side, pathogens on the other. The defense strategy: Wash your hands, keep the germs away. Clean society. There, in a clean society, one knew what made people liable to prosecution. Every individual was responsible for his own morality. Work on self-improvement. Wash your hands, keep the germs away—and you could be squeaky clean. Then, nothing could go wrong. It was the same for the economy. The battle had to be fought against competitors in the market. If you were good, you moved up. If you were bad, you fell down. The bankrupt man was not squeaky clean. It was his own fault, and he was expelled from clean society, either by criminal law or by the economy. Sad as it was, the guilty individual stood alone in the foreground. If you failed, it was your own fault. It was the same way in the battle against the pathogens. If you got sick, it was your own fault. Wash your hands, keep the germs away.

This was plausibility. Since then, it has paled and been replaced by a new plausibility. In retrospect, we sympathize with the skeptics of those times. Before the pathogen comes the opening of the door to the pathogen. And who opens the door? Sometimes the pathogen itself does, if its sheer number renders all resistance useless. Sometimes an individual's carelessness openly invites the pathogen. But there is not always a great number of pathogens or self-culpability. The new plausibility diverted responsibility from the lone individual to "the system." Socialism was victorious after all. Not the way its founders intended. But the fact that we think in big systems, in networks that trap the individual, is the heritage of socialist thinking.

A criminal? It was not his fault! A murderer or a thief? The social environment had failed. A bad system produced a bad person. This must be considered extenuating circumstances. The manager of a bankrupt company? It was not his fault! Thousands of workers forced into unemployment? A result of structural change. No individual can be blamed for that. It is so obvious! A student did not manage to graduate? The poor dear could not cope with the educational system. It is much too elitist. Talents are stifled. Why always study grammar, mathematics, chemistry, and physics? Not everyone needs that stuff. Just opt out of it.

The sick person was doubly victimized by the system. First, the environment made him ill. Ah, times were rosy when stress could plausibly be made responsible for peptic ulcers. Helicobacter was still undiscovered. It was the fault of the economic system, which drove a person to despair, or to a stomach ulcer. Second, the body's defense system has failed. Why? Perhaps because the environment caused so much stress. Perhaps it was this, perhaps it was that. Whatever had plausibility. As long as we think in terms of social and economic systems, we will also view the organism as a system.

78 | AIDS: The Disease That Fits

AIDS is the disease that fits. It unites the germ theory of disease with systems thinking. AIDS could only arise in the late twentieth century. AIDS is the illness that backs up plausibility. A pathogen gets into the body. Sometimes it lies dormant, only to wake many years later. Sometimes it remains awake and starts its work right away. It weakens or destroys the immune system, with fatal consequences—like tuberculosis or other opportunistic diseases. They are parasites, so to speak. They recognize a weak immune system and take advantage of the opportunity. This is AIDS. How did a cynic in the scientific academia put it? *If AIDS hadn't come by itself, it would have been invented.* Indeed, the encounter with HIV/AIDS has showered unprecedented financial resources on virologists' laboratories. Indeed, the encounter with HIV/AIDS has brought tremendous inspiration to virologists' research. What a vast amount we have learned about retroviruses, and in such a short time! Barely twenty years. This is reality. Hats off to the virologists, and Nobel Prizes to the scientists who discovered the virus's secret code. But AIDS?

We could venture a hypothesis: in, say, sixty or perhaps a hundred years, people will shake their heads over the interpretation of AIDS that lasted from 1982 to the early twenty-first century. In retrospect, our era could be thus summarized thus:

> The disease model of HIV/AIDS that emerged in the late twentieth and early twenty-first century—and found broad acceptance in teaching, research, and therapy—was clearly marked by the social and economic circumstances of the time. It had plausibility, but as we know today, it did not correspond with reality. This plausibility gained its persuasiveness through several factors. At its center was systems thinking in economics, criminal law, and many other domains, which had been emerging since the mid-twentieth century.
>
> By the late twentieth century, systems thinking was flanked by a growing consciousness of living in a hitherto intact world, now increasingly threatened by intruders (the benevolent spoke of immigrants and asylum seekers, the less benevolent of illegal aliens and economic migrants). Closed borders or openness to immigration was the big political debate of the time. This fear was mirrored in the HIV/AIDS metaphor, in which an organism whose immune system is weakened by intruders becomes vulnerable to all kinds of trouble and is ultimately killed.
>
> As always in the history of medicine, the organism of the individual human corresponded to the organism of social life. The plausibility of the HIV/AIDS disease model was further nourished by the events of September 11, 2001, when Muslim extremists killed thousands of people in an attack on the World Trade Center in New York. From that time on, terrorists were a generally known and feared phenomenon. A courageous foreign body that followed orders to harm its host organism, whereby the terrorist himself is also destroyed. The United States established the Department of Homeland Security, which one might call the "Department of Strengthening National Immunity" in retrospect. Immune powers were conjured up everywhere. It became law to sort out the good from the bad newcomers at the borders, and to prevent foreign bodies from entering the organism. Efforts were intensified everywhere to find and remove germs that had already entered the organism.
>
> Thus we conclude our retrospective look at the past one hundred years. We have attempted to show the extent to which disease models of the late twentieth and early twenty-first century were marked by the zeitgeist and societal circumstances. Of course, those alive at the time could not realize this. Only today do we know that . . .

Unfortunately, this is a dream of no use to those now suffering from this disease.

Let us summarize again what had happened at the western end of the Eurasian continent: Europeans put their architects and engineers to work for many centuries. They had taken a good look at quite a few masterpieces. They had gone for a while into one cage or another. They had tried out living in the creations, so to speak. Some were very extensive and possessed of many rooms, like Jean Fernel's edifice of ideas. We recall that there was so much spirit and such a short life span. Suddenly the zeitgeist changed, leaving the wrecking ball to tear through mercilessly. For a long time, no one dared to make another attempt.

Finally, in the nineteenth century, a new cage emerged that now included everyone and held all in its grasp. It resulted from the combined powers of many builders. All those searching for a new medicine found themselves in the cage of this new science. They went inside and closed the door. The last one in turned off the light outside. Now the only light was inside. The bars were borrowed from chemistry, physics, and technology, and they stood very close together. Hardly any inmates close to the bars looking out could discern even a pale shimmer. Everyone was inside. The bars were strong and sturdy, imparting safety and stability. The cage itself was illuminated by plausibility. The lamps had names like immunology or the germ theory of disease. Once in a while a light bulb went out, and a new one was put in.

79 | China in the Nineteenth Century: A New Cage Opens Up

This was the medicine that was brought to China at the beginning of the nineteenth century. There, the upper class of Confucian society (about 5 percent of the population) still wandered around in the two-thousand-year-old cage of systematic correspondences. Yet the bars of the brands "yin-yang" or "five agents" were getting rubbery and soft, and the candles of plausibility were almost burnt out. But nothing better was available to provide stability and light. Thus, no one found the way out—until the substitute arrived from the West. The defection from one cage to another happened quickly and without effective resistance. Within a few decades, the new cage had convinced virtually every decision-maker in China.

Let us pause for a moment. It is worth taking a closer look at the convergence of these two traditions. For two millennia, from the first century BC to the nineteenth century, the cultural upper class of Chinese civilization had clung to a medicine that owed its plausibility to the structures of the ancient unification of kingdoms. It equally owed its plausibility to the sociopolitical ideals of Confucian and legalistic social philosophers. We have already spoken of this in detail, when we determined the plausibility that illuminated the birth of this medicine. For the majority of China's intellectual elite, and also for an increasing part of the remaining population, in the nineteenth and twentieth centuries this plausibility was but a distant sunset on the horizon. It had been a long time since it had given light to the seeker.

Over the centuries, the ancient doctrines of social theory had become rigid, their contents reduced to empty clichés. The structures of the ancient empire were now dated. The empire faltered in the nineteenth and fell at the beginning of the twentieth century. Totally new ways of organizing social life were first promoted as ideals and later formed into reality. Seen in retrospect, and in light of the hypothesis advocated here, the customary medical thinking did not have a chance, even for short-term survival. It was as if a tree already weakened by old age was uprooted and deprived of the earth from which it took its strength. So it went with the traditional medicine of China. A few insistent authors' verbose, anachronistic attempt to halt the threatening decline affected nothing but the paper it was printed on.

80 | Two Basic Ideas of Medicine

What about European medicine? How did it affect the Chinese? This seems like only one question when in fact it is two: Did European medicine seem foreign or familiar to the Chinese? Was it useful for treating their illnesses and epidemics? Of course, a few things in the new medicine were foreign, about as foreign as acupuncture was for Europeans. But this was only the surface of things, a matter of technique. Behind that, the underlying ideas were hidden. And these were not foreign at all.

There are two fundamental ideas in medicine—in China as in Europe. Can we separate plausibility and reality? One fundamental idea sees inherent laws in society, nature, and the human body. He who follows the laws survives and stays healthy. He who disobeys the laws will be punished, mildly or harshly, depending on the offense. Sometimes disobedience can cost one's life. This is no different in society than it is in nature. The more civilized a society is, the more it can moderate the extent of punishment. Nature, on the other hand, is always merciless. The task of medicine is to protect people from the merciless punishments of nature.

The other fundamental idea is that plausibility projects social life onto the life of the individual organism: We have friends, but we also have enemies. We must be on guard against our enemies. They can hurt us. There are enemies that wait to attack and then make us waste away, bleed, and perhaps even die. These enemies are visible. They are reality. War is reality. Time and time again.

The individual organism sometimes wastes away without any attack by a visible enemy. In such cases, it must have been a miniscule or invisible enemy. The names for the smallest enemies that could wreak such havoc were different in China and in Europe over the centuries. Xu Dachun was firmly convinced of their existence. So were Fracastoro and Samuel Hahnemann. We cannot be certain what Giovanni Morgagni thought. But Robert Koch convinced all of Europe. At the end of the nineteenth century, Western medicine arrived at the insight that had been present in China for two millennia.

81 | Value-free Biology and Cultural Interpretation

How did Western medicine seem to the Chinese? Not unfamiliar, at least in its fundamental ideas. The powers of self-healing were unknown to them, but this could easily be compensated for. The idea of powers of self-healing had been unwelcome, even in European healing. Patients who believe in powers of self-healing wait too long before seeking treatment. Physicians do not like that very much. The Chinese, influenced by the Confucians' early intervention maxims, did not like that very much either. European physicians were forced into a discussion of this by democrats who believed in the ability of every organism to organize itself. But they did not like it. And they still do not like it, especially today, when the practice of medicine is subject to economic factors. No one wants to lose a patient to the healer in the organism. So the emphasis is on prevention, which usually means early detection (for money) and early treatment (for money). Just as it has been in China for the past two millennia.

We must not forget immunology, molecular biologists' newest playing field. This is a systems thought that has qualified germ theory. It was timely in Europe, corresponding to the socialist thought of the twentieth century. And even this is familiar to the Chinese. It was long known that in the organism, defenders patrol and lie in wait for invaders, fighting defensive battles against them. The ancient Chinese called these defenders *wei*. Literally translated, this means "defense forces." Two millennia ago, this was pure military plausibility, because there was not yet molecular biology that could have published this plausibility as a scientific insight. Plausibility illuminated the functions in the body's interior.

Let us not misunderstand each other: the immune reaction is not mere plausibility, it is reality. The reality is that there are antigens that the organism recognizes as foreign to the body, which can cause the creation of antibodies. The reality is that specific antibodies are formed and secreted only after invasion by a certain antigen. The reality is that the antibodies occasionally also wrongly identify other antibodies, made by the same organism, as foreign to the body. It is reality that the antigen-antibody reaction can result in the formation of immune complexes that are no longer soluble, that precipitate and are taken up and digested by phagocytes. The reality is that there are soluble immune complexes that can invade and trigger harmful mechanisms in vessels and tissues. The reality is that very small or very large amounts of antigens cause no immune reaction.

Reality becomes plausibility if the antigen is interpreted as an invader in the social or military sense. It is that simple. There is no enmity between foreign and endogenic substances. There are merely value-neutral biological reactions between various biochemical substances. Nothing more. Enmity is a value judgment, made by people in a certain cultural context, because humans create "their" medicine in accordance with their values, in order to survive as long as they can. This requires making judgments. But nature knows no such judgments. There is no enmity between antigen and organism. The antigen is part of nature. The antibody is part of nature. Their meeting is a reaction that in many cases leads to the formation of a reaction product that in turn serves as nourishment for other cells. How nice for the other cells. We call them phagocytes. Sometimes, the organism does not react to foreign substances. That is how it developed in nature, the result of a higher equilibrium that humans cannot grasp in all its details. But we would like to influence it in a way that makes it useful for our survival. Hence the value judgment of the involved components. Hence the plausibility of the enmity ideas, of the military ideas.

The culture of medicine takes certain processes out of value-neutral biology and judges them. It did so two millennia ago in China, without knowledge of the initial phase and the effectual phase, of anaphylactic, cytotoxic, or cell-mediated reaction. It does so today, in modern medicine. Knowledge of reality has changed considerably. Yet the cultural interpretation has stayed the same. How did European medicine seem to the Chinese? Not unfamiliar, at least in its fundamental ideas. The Chinese had simply been two millennia ahead of their time!

82 | A Transit Visa and a Promise

And how did it seem in practice? What did it have to offer in the nineteenth and early twentieth century? The medicine of Europe was still in a transitional stage. It was a transit visa for the present, with the promise of a golden future. This was what made the new medicine appear so interesting. Not only in Europe, but, after the 1860s, also in Japan. And now, in China! The new medicine received this transit visa for the present with the promise of a golden future partly because of the environment it grew out of. This environment was marked by technology and the new natural sciences, whose proximity physicians sought. The successes of this technology were unmistakably clear and, above all, interculturally applicable everywhere in the world, including China.

The new medicine also received this transit visa because of a breathtaking production of successes of its own. These successes were also reality: unmistakable and above all interculturally evident. The increasingly detailed exact knowledge of the interior of the body and surgery, the knowledge of the pathogens and the successful struggle to control epidemics. This was not mere plausibility, but reality. For millennia, the Chinese—officials in the city and peasants in the countryside—had nothing better to fight plagues with than magic and rituals. So these methods were used to attempt to expel plague demons, even as late as in the nineteenth century. When, in 1910, a great plague afflicted Manchuria, it was the Western-trained bacteriologist Wu Lien-Teh who effectively challenged magic rituals and showed them the door. This was convincing. For those with eyes to see and ears to hear, there was no doubt: only Western medicine could bring China, "the sick man," to strength again.

After initial wavering about whether the old cage could be lent stability through the exchange of some cage bars, discussion since the beginning of the twentieth century has concentrated on one question above all: Is it possible to link the two cages? The old cage had done well for a long time, providing security and stability. Could not the two be placed side by side? This was the central question that arose. Opinions are divided on this question. First in China, later also in the West. But each in its own time.

83 | Scorn, Mockery, and Invectives for Chinese Medicine

In 1835, Peter Parker (1804–1888), an American missionary and physician, opened an ophthalmologic practice in Canton. The American Board of Commissioners for Foreign Missions had sent Peter Parker to save the souls of the Chinese. After a short introduction to his host country, he preferred to concentrate on saving their bodies, especially their eyes. There was a lot to do. Peter Parker did not have many practical tools in his bag that were superior to the healing of the Chinese. But his surgery was vastly different from anything in China. His interventions in the eye were extremely impressive. People lined up to see him. Peter Parker gave out numbers in an attempt to order the crowds. Soon, more medically trained missionaries came and lured the Chinese into their practices with the prospect of treatment of physical ills. They hoped to reroute them from there into their churches. Soon, the first Chinese were venturing to the United States to study this new medicine at its source.

In the mid-1850s, the Briton Benjamin Hobson wrote a multivolume introduction to Western science and medicine. Guan Maocai helped him translate it into Chinese. Hobson depicted a steam locomotive for the first time. He was the first to offer views into the interior of the body, never seen by the Chinese in such distinctness. He explained operations and the related instruments. All of this was previously unknown in China, yet it was immediately convincing. The medicine that used modern technology must be just as successful as modern technology. Putting airplanes into the sky was still to come. But military technology on land and sea had already made a great impression. And the locomotive was visible to all. Even if some peasants in the villages opposed the railroad, the medicine that appeared with this technology had to be just as successful.

Hobson saw a fundamental difference and described it in his introduction for the Chinese readers: In Europe, research is done, because true knowledge lies in the future. In China, no research is done, because perfect knowledge is already available in ancient books. This was not completely true, but it captured the general tendencies. Europe's unbelievable enthusiasm in the nineteenth and early twentieth century to gain new knowledge by doing research and experiments had no parallel in China's own tradition. The cage of systematic correspondences had not yet opened up. And within that cage, no research could be established.

Something had to change: this was clear to Chinese intellectuals by the end of the nineteenth century. The early attempt to buy certain Western technologies and use them for defense against the West failed miserably. The imperial system had reached its end. Two millennia of Chinese cultural tradition had reached their end. Thus, an ever greater number of Chinese reformers emerged. The Middle Kingdom was no longer a kingdom, nor was it in the middle. Countless associations of worried patriots were founded, where people thought about things, invited the most important Western thinkers, and asked them and themselves about the reasons for Western strength.

The peak of this search came during and after World War I, when the imperial powers humiliated China. The decision to now uncompromisingly accept Western science and technology was brutal, but unavoidable. There was no difference of opinion on this between nationalists and communists. Western medicine went along with Western science. What scorn, what mockery, what invectives poured out of the reformers onto the Chinese healing tradition. Several authors and filmmakers at this time of awakening used Chinese medicine as a symbol of their fathers' and grandfathers' most decadent ways of thinking and put Chinese medicine at the center of their attacks on the structures that were now to be overcome. At the end of the 1920s, an impetuous and un-Chinese petition for a referendum was introduced to completely forbid tradition, effective immediately. It failed due to the resistance of vested interests, the chaotic domestic political situation during the civil war, and the Japanese invasion, but that did not help much. The decision-makers, the reformers, trusted solely in modern Western medicine. They accused their own tradition of being partly responsible for China's illness.

84 | Traditional Medicine in the PRC: Faith in Science

With the victory of the People's Liberation Army and the founding of the People's Republic of China (PRC) in 1949, Marxists made a decision about the future of medicine—adapted to the situation in China according to the thoughts of Mao. Since then, authorities have proceeded skillfully. The heritage of traditional medicine is cited, praised as the legacy of the people, and then undermined from the inside out. The roots and earth from which the tradition once pulled its strength were long since taken from the tree. But what was to be done with all that wood? Healers were still carving successful therapies out of it! But the interpretation was missing, which is not an easy thing to provide.

Compromises had to be made. Memories of the old doctrines of yin-yang and the five agents were kept alive—but from a distance! They were relativized as attempts of the ancestors to master the powers of nature with materialistic thinking. These were primitive attempts, but still attempts to leave behind the numinous and metaphysical, and to open oneself to materialism. The time of these attempts has passed. Marxism, regardless of its strain, trusts only modern science, pointing to the future. If science cannot explain everything today, then tomorrow or someday later it will. But that is still the goal one must aim for and slowly steer toward. And this is precisely the policy of the People's Republic of China.

The old cage has opened up. From 1950 to 1975, commissions gutted the theoretical edifice and totally rebuilt it from the inside: set pieces from the past were put together carefully so that they no longer clashed with the new knowledge, with the reality of the new Western medicine.[86] The new building corresponds to modern thinking in its internal logic. The old, typically Chinese inductive thinking was exchanged for modern logic, the Western way of thinking. The great, multiroomed, confusing, two-millennia-old cage of ideas was now turned into a cute little playpen, where nobody could get lost anymore. It was easy to handle. Tens of thousands of book chapters of heterogeneous contents, millions of knowledge-filled pages, now condensed into "overviews"—booklets barely one or two centimeters thick. This is what remains of the theories of Chinese traditional medicine, after the lights that had conferred plausibility to them for two millennia were extinguished.

85 | The Arabs of the Twentieth Century, or Crowding in the Playpen

Yet the saviors are already close by: the "Arabs" of the twentieth and twenty-first century. The plausibility of the old Greek medicine had paled following the end of the Roman Empire in the Early Middle Ages. The Arabs emerged from the desert, and in Aleppo and elsewhere were introduced to what the Christian West no longer wanted. The Arabs were rightly astonished. The knowledge was foreign to them. It seemed incomprehensibly superior to their own healing practices. They translated, compiled, and became the preservers of an ancient inheritance that was spurned by the Christians themselves. Of course, they were only preservers, admirers, and users of this inheritance. Their situation and environment was not suited to breathe new life and new thoughts into the old medicine. But nevertheless, great names are connected with this preserving, admiring, and using: Hunayn ibn Ishaq (alias Johannitius, 808–873), Abu Bakr Muhammed ibn Zakariya ar-Razi (alias Rhazes, 865–925), Abu al-Qasim Khalaf ibn al-Abbas al-Zahrawi (alias Abulcasis, 939–1010), Abu Ali ibn Sina (alias Avicenna, 980–1037), and many others will eternally be remembered as the saviors who sheltered the ancient medicine until the Christian West remembered it again.

We are now witness to a similar process. In China, traditional medicine is now officially only valid in playpen format. It was, of course, only intended for temporary use. One grows out of it. What the Chinese had not expected was crowding in the playpen. They had hardly opened their doors to the West, first hesitantly in the mid-1970s and then enthusiastically in 1978 (following Richard Nixon's handshake), before it got crowded in the cute little playpen; crowded with the immense masses of those whom the Chinese, in complete ignorance of the Western state of mind, had imagined to be disciples of pure scientific teaching. The European and American Arabs had arrived. With incredible astonishment, they learned about needle treatments, herbal knowledge, and summaries of the doctrines.

On the Chinese side, the situation was swiftly recognized. A new product, designed by the commission, received a name in its own language: *zhongyi* (Chinese medicine), in contrast to *xiyi* (Western medicine). An English term was also coined to be used by the ignorant Arabs from the cultural desert of the West: Traditional Chinese Medicine. This name was misleading and led the visitors truly astray. There they sat, crowded into the playpen. They felt comfortable, because on the one hand, the playpen had the exotic cage bars of yin-yang and the five agents, and, on the other hand, it was also very familiar. It was easy to learn.

And this is what the visitors took in thin booklets back home, where they happily proclaimed that they now possessed the knowledge of a several-thousand-year-old culture. Soon, the "Abus" and "Ibns" of Europe and North America emerged. From the thin booklets, books of many hundred pages were written. First a few, then increasingly more. Key words were flourished like banners before the eyes of the surprised masses at home: Holism! Nature! Energy! Inductive synthesis, not causal analysis! Every returnee built a small playpen at home, based on the model. The blueprint was easy to learn. Some stayed only one or two weeks in the original land. Others spent somewhat more time. Still others did not journey there at all, but just listened in to the secrets of the returnees. And each one built a private playpen. In the United States, England, France, Germany and Italy. But the copies did not completely work. They did not really want to look Chinese, and the building materials were more Western. But the set pieces brought from China were enough to confer a taste of the Far East.

86 ⎪ When the Light Comes from Behind

The avalanche had begun. Just twenty years later, there was hardly a town in the Western world that had not heard the Good News. The Arabs did their duty: they became admirers of an ancient heritage whose people were trying to leave it behind. Of course, among the "Abus" and "Ibns" of Europe and North America, there were some who looked closely and recognized the fraud. They realized that this Traditional Chinese Medicine, often known by its trade logo TCM, was not identical with actual Chinese traditional medicine, and so they set to work. They wanted to be protectors, admirers, and users, but not of a new, hollow product painted onto a canvas of Western logic. No, it should be the true doctrine: the Classics. And so an effort was started to call a stop to the tendency in China. A lot was at stake. The true heritage, and how this true heritage should be defended, was the topic of *German Sermons on Chinese Medicine*.[87]

One of the involuntary addressees of these *German Sermons* was State President Jiang Zemin. He was quite surprised, in the year 2001, to receive a letter from Germany promising him a lot of money if he, the president, would ensure that the adopted course would be left and the real, classical medicine of China would be helped to a renaissance—in

China, with the guidance of the German lecturer. Well, after appraisal by the relevant institutions, the letter was filed away with much head shaking, along with other documents of unwelcome foreign interference. But it nevertheless shows one thing: the Arabs have made a comeback, even if today they are European and no longer need an alias.

Interesting, isn't it? The moment the Chinese open their doors, seeking a serious change in direction toward the future, droves of men and women flock to China from the future-oriented civilization of the West with the wish to learn—not of the adaptation to the present, but of the classics of antiquity. The cultures have met at a crossroads. On the one side are those who have decided, after slowly walking forward with their heads turned backward for two millennia, to turn their heads around and look forward. They are met by those who were educated to look forward but are walking backward. A very nice picture. But that's exactly how it is.

It is possible to walk forward while facing backward—when the light comes from behind. For centuries in the European history of ideas, apart from the light of religious promise, aspirations were aimed at the bright sun of ever more complete knowledge in the future. Why look back? The historian is an exception. But otherwise? Only obsolete knowledge can be found in the past. So it is better to turn to the future! But now, for part of the Western population, the light again comes from the past. It says: Turn around and continue to march while facing backward—and always keep the light in view. This light gives off a warm, mild glow. Let us call this light, since we have already encountered it so often, plausibility.

87 | In the Beginning Was the Word

Now we must repeat questions we asked above. How did TCM affect the citizens of industrialized Western nations—their minds and their bodies? We can answer both questions with one word: promising! First came the effect on the mind. It was promising. That was no different from other big innovations in the theory of medicine. First, theories had to affect the mind. They had to be promising. We have met the exceptions: John Brown and his medicine of opium, alcohol, and spices. He felt the effects on his own body before he clothed them in theoretical explanations. Franz Anton Mesmer, who first healed Fräulein Oester-lin with magnets and only then developed his theory. Finally, there is Samuel Hahnemann. Never before and never again has a physician so long experimented and thought things over before fitting his rather acci-dental clinical observations onto a theoretical edifice. These are the three exceptions. But they are not the rule; the rule is different.

In the beginning there was the Word. The Word possesses plausibility and persuasiveness. And why does the Word possess plausibility and persuasiveness? Because it mirrors experiences and visions. Because it mirrors the real or ideal structures that humans live in or would like to live in. Because it mirrors existential fears, and the supposedly appropri-ate strategies for overcoming those fears. When a medicine was first cre-ated in Greek and then in Chinese antiquity, the experiences and visions of both civilizations—the real and ideal structures, the fears and strate-gies to escape them—were funneled into these two completely new are-nas of healing. Starting in the 1970s, something different was happening in Europe and North America: The entire Western world had common experiences and visions, real and ideal structures, as well as fears and corresponding strategies—but its medicine was no longer appropriate for them. At least for part of the population.

88 | Out of Touch with Nature

A new era was dawning. The terrible suspicion arose that chemistry, physics, and technology were no longer suitable for solving the present problems of humanity. The first energy crises made a deep impression and were etched into people's memories. Sufficient sources of energy were available: but were they safe? Two great, hitherto unknown fears crept into Western souls. On the one hand, there was a fear of a more destructive power of chemistry, physics, and technology. Three Mile Island, Bhopal, Seveso—these were the first signs of these new dangers. Many more followed. "Nature," for millennia the adversary of humanity from which we had to protect ourselves, became the victim of human actions, worthy of protection.

The word *nature* does ridiculously poor justice to the idea of nature. Nature cannot be destroyed by humanity. Nature will always be superior; it will always prevail. Not the other way around. It would be more suitable to say that humans, under the spell of chemistry, physics, and technology, have fallen out of touch with nature and forgotten how to restrain our overconfidence. The result is not the destruction of nature. The result is the exact opposite. Nature is irritated, and stirred up in her powers to such a degree that she will certainly destroy those who endeavored to escape her powers, or even wanted to befriend her. "An unspeakable entity, our friend, rules over things. Everything that nature creates is both perfect and beautiful. One credits nature with being the highest authority on reason and with the ability to be beautiful."[88] And people want to be able to destroy that? Ridiculous. We cannot destroy nature. We can destroy the basis for our livelihood by setting powers free *in* nature that we can no longer restrain. The destruction of nature is not humanity's destruction of nature. The destruction of nature is nature's destruction of humanity, the same nature we believed we could control.

The certainty of the impending destruction of nature scares us. This is not what we had in mind. It should be the reverse. We are the ruler of nature. But it has happened differently. Nature is the ruler of humankind. This is frightening. The new worship of nature is nothing other than secular idolatry. People in industrialized nations have unleashed a wild force and are now trying to tame that force. We will not succeed, but fears nevertheless compel people to try. Not everyone, at least not yet, but increasingly more people. Where to begin with the taming? With one's self. That is something that can perhaps be controlled—simply no longer allow things that might further irritate nature to come near or into one's body.

Chemotherapy? Medication from basic chemical materials? Chemical preservatives in marmalade? Simply no longer allow them into the body. This helps allay fears that one could offend or irritate nature even more, maybe even to the point that she takes one's body away. Chemistry offends nature. So chemistry is to be avoided. Idolatry. Sacrifices have to be made. Chinese medicine came along at just the right time. It uses herbs; it uses needles that are removed from the body after treatment. This is natural. This was offered to nature, as naturopathy. For appeasement.

"Dear nature, I promise not to ingest any more chemicals into myself/ into you. In return, please keep me from getting sick." If only it were so simple. Seldom has a confusion of ideas been greater. But the prayer helped, because it allayed the fears. If naturopathy is really supposed to stand at the center of the new idolatry, so be it: water, warmth, heat, light, and air are natural. To let them take their effects on the body is beneficial in many respects, economical, tried and tested. But this was not the point. The idolatry of "nature" required a theology, and this was certainly not offered by the use of water, warmth, heat, light, and air. This is too primitive. So-called Chinese medicine was better equipped to provide the required theology. It simultaneously presented itself as a secularized religion.

89 | Theology without *Theos*

Conventional religion gives meaning and answers questions: Why do I exist? What is my relationship to the universe? How should I live? Who created me? What will happen in the future? Religion is also the integration of the individual into the greater whole. Most people wish for this integration and ask the above questions. In the past, answers were given in church. But with the anxieties arising from modern challenges, such as the energy crisis, environmental pollution, and an increasingly impersonal, technology based medicine, ever more people seek answers elsewhere. The "theology" of Chinese medicine gives answers that believers in the churches of conventional religion have to live without.

Of course, this "theology" is not theology, because it has no *theos*. The yin-yang and five agents doctrines are the cosmology of a secular religion. It is a religion, because it makes the individual's integration in the greater whole understandable. It is secular, because the numinous does not exist in this religion. No god or gods. No demons or ancestors. He who is bothered by such ideas in conventional theologies can now turn to the new cosmology. The churches become superfluous. Yin-yang and the five agents answer all the central questions: Why do I exist? What is my relationship to the universe? How should I live? Who created me? What will happen in the future? How am I integrated into the greater whole?

One can start with one's self, or do one's best to help the greater whole. Following the yin-yang and five agents doctrines, this comprises the new morality. He who acts immorally sins against his body on a small scale, or against the universe on a large scale. The idea of sin is common to secular and church religions. But they have something else in common: for two millennia, Westerners have heard the optimistic message of hope, of confidence. We are used to this. We want to be able to hope, to have confidence: everything will be fine. This hope is also found in the new, secular religion of the East. The cyclical ideas of yin-yang and the five agents promise hope. This hope is much needed in a time when the media report bad news daily. With increasingly more chemistry, technology, and energy requirements—how can the environment ever recover?

90 | Everything Will Be Fine

Even half a century ago, there was a single dominant attitude toward life: it will always keep improving. With chemistry, physics, and technology, everything will become easier, more beautiful, simpler. But then there was an upheaval sometime in the 1970s. An increasing number of citizens of industrialized Western nations believed that chemistry, physics, and technology would cause everything to break down, get uglier, and become more difficult. Everything is heading downhill, with a final catastrophe in view. Not everyone shared this grim way of thinking. But increasing numbers of people no longer found comfort and hope in the Church. There, no one took a stand against the destruction of the environment. The Club of Rome was very close to the Vatican. But the Vatican was very far from the Club of Rome. Did priests and theologians take to the streets to protest Seveso and Bhopal? No one had seen or heard any protest from them. People had, in the meantime, started getting their answers elsewhere, at a place where hope is subliminally delivered with the rest of the order: cyclical thinking promises a return to the starting point.

Anyone interested can investigate the details. When, for example, the wood phase becomes too overpowering, it threatens the earth phase. Wood perforates earth. Too much wood takes strength from the earth. Too many trees on a dam remove its strength to actually dam the water. Yet, all by itself, the overconfidence of the wood phase awakens counteracting forces. The metal phase is the child of the earth phase. The metal phase sees his mother, the earth phase, in danger. Metal can cut wood down to size. And this is what happens. The wood phase is cut down to size by the metal phase. Thus, it loses its power to perforate the earth. The earth is no longer threatened by any danger. Metal, son of earth, can calm down, since no danger is threatening his mother any longer. The earth can now strengthen herself again. Everything is fine.

91 | Left Alone in the Computer Tomograph

Along with chemistry, physics and technology were also sacrificed at the altar of the new idolatry. Let us remember when highways and mobility were praised and extolled, day after day, summer and winter. It was considered a blessing to be linked with faraway places. And now, the new era. The thing that connects also divides, because to be created it had to destroy. The focus shifted from the connecting function of highways and automobiles to their destructiveness. Destroyed landscapes, poisoned air. People feared many of the outward manifestations of modern technology, including medicine.

Modern medicine uses technology, even nuclear technology, in diagnosis and therapy. But not only this. Technology comes between physician and patient. In diagnosis, the patient is examined by technology—perhaps even left alone in a computer tomograph. Test results are transmitted to invisible technologists and physicians via monitors. They compare the results with cold data, maybe while chatting about their vacation, a new

car, their girlfriend. They determine deviations from the norm on print-
outs and monitors. This is a tremendous advance in the treatment of the
sick—but, nevertheless, it is frightening. Not to everyone, but to many
people. They miss having a physician who personally examines, palpates,
talks to them, treats them with his or her hands, and considers their personal fate. The image of high-tech medicine overlaid the successes of this
medicine, creating fears that pushed people to seek alternatives. TCM was
such an alternative. Acupuncture promised that no technology would
come between physician and patient. Instead, there would be direct touch:
a needle that leaves no chemical residues behind. This was reassuring.

92 | Healing and the Energy Crisis

How did TCM affect the citizens of industrialized Western nations? It
was reassuring to the fearful soul. Modern medicine was missing something: the belief in a life force. It is not measurable, not perceptible, and
therefore it evades the search for reality. Airplanes in the sky and bridges
over straits—no life force is needed for that. Chemistry, physics, and
technology are enough. One of the European saviors of TCM expressed
it thus:

> The existence of a life force is ignored by Western science. The life force,
> life vitality, is central to the understanding of life processes in 106 cultures
> worldwide. Yet it has been lost in the development of Western medicine over
> the past one hundred years. . . . The flowing life force, the Chinese *qi*, in
> India *prana*, is viewed to be the source of all life, and it forms the basis of the
> Chinese description of nature. Qi is life, constantly in motion, flowing, bring-
> ing change. It is present everywhere in nature; it is the life force that shows
> itself in the function and movement of everything living. Any stagnation of
> the flowing life energy leads to the disturbance of life processes, and thus
> to disease. Western science cannot measure the life force with instruments,
> therefore it does not exist. . . . So Western scientists . . . have a lot of catching
> up to do.[89]

An attempt, it seems, to introduce back into healing the X, which we
met right at the beginning and whose removal from medicine Virchow
spent his life advocating. And the author was hardly an amateur. He is

in fact highly educated, having successfully completed his studies at a faculty of medicine. He is one of many such advocates.

X has different names in their world image; some we have known since antiquity, some were named for us by Virchow, and more were added: life force, life vitality, flowing life force, qi, prana, life, life energy. It is correct that Western science cannot find any use for these ideas—even with this increased number. But a lot of catching up to do? There is no need for any catching up. Malaria and femoral neck fractures can be treated very well without X; everything else is a private matter. Every group, every individual is free to interpret X as he or she wants. It is also permissible to interpret qi as life energy. This is new and interesting to the Chinese. They did not realize this for two millennia. Now a few Westerners have come along and let them know: qi is life energy. The Chinese were so happy to finally find that out from the West, which was having an energy crisis.

How did TCM affect the citizens of industrialized Western nations? It was reassuring. These citizens—at least a part of them—were troubled by several fears. One of the central, most profound fear-provoking experiences of the 1970s to 1990s was the energy crisis. Parallel to the gradual rapprochement of East and West, it replaced the fear of nuclear war. The energy crisis led to wars in distant lands. In Germany, it led to civil-war-like domestic conflicts over the storage and transport of nuclear waste: battles every evening on the television screen in every living room. This was alarming. It was reassuring to have someone finally pay attention to energy, life energy. A healing dedicated to energy. That was convincing and reassuring. If the conflicts over energy cannot yet be solved in distant lands, then at least they can be solved in my own body. It is a start, at least. Here, I have control. Here, I can begin: nature, not chemicals; intimacy, not technology. Care for life, not civil war.

93 | TCM: Western Fears, Chinese Set Pieces

TCM had a reassuring affect. It allayed fears. These were mainly Western fears. Where did TCM come from? China. Some of it also came from

Japan and Korea. Who wrote and writes the successful books on TCM for a Western audience? The "Abus" and "Ibns." Their names are Ted Kaptchuk, Manfred Porkert, Dan Bensky, Bob Flaws, Jack Worsley, Yves Requena, Père Larre, Joe Helms, Giovanni Maciocia . . . But why is there no Chinese author in this list of bestselling writers? Some have tried it, but they can't seem to reach a large audience. This should astonish us. When Japan decided to adopt Western medicine in the course of the Meiji reforms of the 1860s, German physicians were invited. They enjoyed high status in Japan and were honored as teachers. Their names were the talk of the town. At least until the Japanese caught up with their teachers and became their equals.

The adoption of TCM came about differently. This was because it was not an adoption at all. Rather, it was the creation of a new healing that built upon Western fears and used Chinese set pieces. The Chinese were needed as technicians in Western private clinics. There, they were skilful helpers. They knew how to use needles. But in the big picture? The fears of the citizens of industrialized Western nations were foreign to them. Tailoring so-called Chinese medicine to these fears is something they could not and cannot manage. That we would rather do ourselves.

Here we need to do a bit of polishing. TCM is nice, friendly, soft medicine. Western science has produced a terrible, dangerous, and, at times, deadly medicine. "Abu" and "Ibn" report 106,000 iatrogenic deaths in the United States per year, and then set the gentle TCM next to it.[90] Well, it's true that acupuncture rarely has victims to grieve. Pneumothorax is rare, and so is the broken needle. But the comparison doesn't work. If we are going to make such a comparison, then we should aim to compare apples with apples. Not apples with lychees. Chinese medicine also has its victims. Some lie far in the past. For example, the countless people who trusted the famous poet Su Dongpo (1036–1101), who had lent his honorable name to a prescription recipe. They swallowed his remedy, then died miserably due to the drug's toxicity. Other victims are closer to us.

How convenient that such an exact counting of the victims of the side effects of physician-prescribed medications can only be undertaken in the United States: 106,000. How convenient that for China, we only can

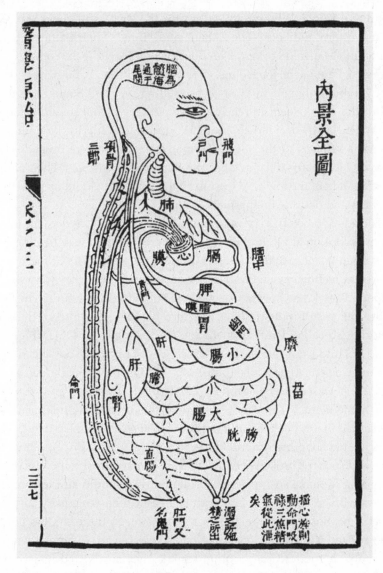

Figure 4. The interior of the human body. From Wang Honghan, Yixue yuanshi, ca. 1722.

suspect how many people are harmed by so-called natural herbs whose contamination with pesticides, herbicides, heavy metals, and benzene still cause Japanese importers to reject up to 80 percent of an import batch. How convenient that we have only a rough idea of how many people were gravely harmed by the improper dosage of aconite. It is more well known that certain plant combinations activate the Epstein-Barr virus to such an extent that this is likely responsible for the high incidence of cancer of the larynx in southern China. But this is never mentioned in the same sentence as the 106,000 victims of Western medicine. Yet we'd have to add a zero or two to that figure. A bit of polishing needs to be done for TCM to be effective and seem reassuring. In the end, we want nature, not chemicals; intimacy, not technology; life energy, not one-sided treatment with medication. And also harmony, not war.

Chinese authors had perhaps not really recognized this. TCM was not allowed to use any warlike vocabulary. After all, it was supposed to allay fears. Warlike vocabulary had been established in the foreground of Chinese medical terminology for two millennia. Even today, it can be found there. But not in Western authors' writings about TCM for Western readers. Their message: a doctrine of peace and harmony. War in our bodies? Modern immunology offered enough of that. Not so much by the immunologists themselves, but by their interpreters: science journalists.

In the influential magazine *Time*, a headline on May 23, 1988, read *Biological Warfare*. That sure got people's attention! The text begins: "The body is constantly being bombarded by viruses, bacteria, and other microbes. When the body is invaded, the microbe begins its attack by multiplying. Within minutes, the immune system, sensing the invader's presence, sends out its forces." And so on. The German media did not want to be upstaged. On October 13, 1987, the Munich daily *Abendzeitung* reported on the Japanese immunologist and Nobel Prize winner Susumo Tonegawa, "the man who unraveled the mystery of the war in our bodies." On March 13, 1995, the weekly magazine *Focus* reported "daily massacres" of "horrifying carnage," and "secret acts of sabotage, hidden allies, and the search for a magic weapon." The message is rounded out by many other similarly worded media reports from the front.

Patients have a choice. A woman who has breast cancer and needs to take chemo can allow an oncologist to explain the war in her own body. That makes you tough. You have to mentally take sides and then the battle really gets going. There is collateral damage; victory is not certain. "Fought the battle and lost," is the message we find in the death announcements of those who did not make it.

The alternative? Restore harmony in the organism. Settle imbalances. Balance yin and yang. Nourish deficiencies. Who could argue with that? For most people, the encounter with a potentially fatal illness is the most existential threat there is. In this situation, who wants their own body to be transformed into a battlefield with an unknown outcome and collateral damage? You can watch that on television. No one wants to experience war in their own house, much less in their own body. At a time of existential fear, we want to feel warmth, empathy, and harmony. This is what TCM offers. It seems reassuring. At least in the polished version, without the traditional military metaphors.

94 | Harmony, Not War

How did TCM seem to the citizens of industrialized Western nations? It seemed reassuring. We were worried by many things, like the "loss of the center." Hans Sedlmayr lamented this in art in 1948. Picasso is an example: "In Picasso, we see the process of division, the Cubist division of the intact human form into layers, its fragmentation into constituent parts, so that one is thrust into the deep to seek the elementary archetypes that man consists of."[91] Berdayev, whom Sedlmayr quotes here, was discussing art. And yet, the same could also be said about medicine. Among the accusations of those who despair of modern medicine, we find dehumanization, antihumanism, detachment from the human, reduction to the inorganic, and many more of Sedlmayr's key words.

The loss of the center is also, above all, the loss of central meaning. In daily life, the meaning that religion imparted for centuries is no longer accepted. In medical practice, the meaning of being ill does not have a code in physicians' billing systems. How and where one is sick, what lab values are elevated, what tissues damaged, what genes mutated, all this can be learned by going to the doctor. But the meaning behind it? The Why? You can't find that out. Reality knows no meaning. Reality is simply there. Meaning is interpretation. Interpretation is a private matter. Many people are still not used to that. They want to have the interpretation delivered with the rest of the order. They want more than just reality. They want to know the original source of their illness. Modern medicine cannot do that. It is not allowed to, since it is based on the laws of nature, which have no meaning. They are simply there, as they are.

TCM offers a center. It offers meaning. It rejects the inorganic and centers on the life force, qi. It links various complaints and traces them back to one central illness. It names this central illness something like kidney-yang weakness and hints that it can be regulated. This gives meaning to the illness and promises a return into the greater balance—without chemicals, without technology in diagnosis and therapy, without warfare or the certainty of collateral damages. It seems reassuring.

95 | The Loss of the Center

How does TCM affect the citizens of industrialized Western nations? It affects not only the mind. It also affects the body, in a very concrete way. It eliminates pain and some other afflictions. It produces contented patients and contented healers. But that came later. In the beginning was the Word, that is, theory. Theory had the glow of plausibility. It lured the citizens of industrialized Western nations, even before it seemed everyone had a neighbor, sister, or colleague who knew someone it actually helped. The Word alone seemed reassuring to the mind, because it spoke to so many fears.

The effects on the body came later—unavoidably, as for the past two millennia. First Asclepiades and Athenaios, later Hildegard von Bingen, Paracelsus, van Helmont, John Brown, Franz Anton Mesmer, Samuel Hahnemann, Friedrich Hoffmann, and so many others. They all had happy, contented patients. They basked in the limelight of their therapeutic successes—just as long as it was not a femoral neck fracture, breast cancer, or malaria. Not then, but with most day-to-day illnesses. It is the same with

TCM. Who could doubt it? To statistically analyze it would be a waste of time. We believe it even without analysis. Because for us this is about theory, the Word. TCM was also about the Word in the beginning, and it was effective, convincing, and reassuring. Clinical success came later. It was inevitable, one might say.

96 | Contented Customers in a Supermarket of Possibilities

This is the astonishing thing. Modern Western medicine works for the Chinese. TCM works for the citizens of industrialized Western nations. A cultural exchange—unplanned, yet complete. China had happily exchanged the cage of the systematic correspondences for the cage of modern science. Whoever wants to can still restore the old cage. This is increasingly difficult to do, since hardly anyone knows the original blueprint any more. In the West, those who could not accept the bars of chemistry, physics, and technology constructed the playpen of TCM. Not very original, but at least it can serve as a bucolic healing vacation home, a place to take a rest from the harsh world of science and technology. If things get really serious, one can always quickly head back into the safe cage, which has its extensions everywhere. It comes down to finding the right mix. Sometimes people look for protection here, sometimes there. This way, one can perhaps avoid becoming one of the 106,000 collateral victims of pharmacologically unpracticed physicians.

We have devoted much space to TCM here. This is because TCM deserves to be looked at in so much detail; for a couple of decades, starting in the 1970s, it was in keeping with the times—it spoke to contemporary fears. It is not the only alternative to orthodox medicine. Homeopathy, anthroposophy, Tibetan medicine, Hawaiian spiritual healers, Paracelsian spagyrics, Bach flower remedies, and many other methods restore the sick to health and convey certainty to healers that they have finally found the right treatment. This is a good thing. This is the way it should be in modern society: a supermarket of possibilities. For computers, we have the choice of conventional European suppliers like Siemens, American products from Hewlett Packard, and Asian products from

Toshiba. For a philosophy of life, we have the choice of conventional European suppliers like the Christian churches, American products like Scientology, and Asian products like Zen Buddhism. The same is true for healing: we have the choice of conventional orthodox medicine and alternatives from Europe, TCM and Ayurveda from Asia, and molecular biology from the New World.

In this supermarket of possibilities, customers still spend the most money on products from Europe and North America. In the end, the reconstructed TCM playpen is also a Western product. But it is certainly not mainstream. German health insurance plans spend an estimated half billion euros on acupuncture, which is not much, considering the total spending of about 180 billion euros in the health system. It is unlikely to increase. The TCM doctrine is no longer in keeping with the times. The initial plausibility of its theory guaranteed its acceptance. For some time now, a transformation to convention has been taking place. Schools instruct practitioners. Effects are seen. Recommendations bring new clients. Profits are made. It is no longer a matter of modest sums. Should the practitioners have to earn their knowledge in 360 compulsory off-campus training hours, or would 140 hours be enough, or perhaps only two or three weekend courses? This is what the debate is about today. Everything else is already routine, convention. Various specialty societies, based on personal experiences and interests, compete and form alliances, depending on the political requirements. This will remain a playpen, where nostalgics say farewell and the usual clientele stops by when it seems opportune. Today's acupuncture needles, tailored to Western sensibilities, are coated with silicone.

97 | The More Things Change

The real money is now flowing elsewhere, because there is change in the air. And where change is in the air, a new medicine also forms. The change can be real, or it can merely play itself out in people's heads. It doesn't necessarily pull the entire population with it. But part of it, a substantial part. Another part clings to the preexisting and doesn't risk change. These are the nostalgics. They are provided for. They can feel safe inside the cage of convention and yell out their horror from within. What is so horrifying? The momentum of molecular, biological medicine. With this we are in the present. Is it possible to observe the present, or even to define it? The way we observe the polis democracy, two millennia ago, or Chinese antiquity? Is it possible to interpret the relationships and cognitive dynamics of the present from a proper distance?

The present is like standing with your nose up against a giant billboard. The billboard is big enough to be seen from a distance, so its message can be understood from a distance. The billboards of the polis democracy and Chinese antiquity are so far away that we believe we can recognize all their essential contours—even if the small print remains obscure. But now we are standing directly in front of today's message, touching the picture with our noses. Is the picture even recognizable? Or must we wait until it slowly distances itself from us, to get the right measures of detailed knowledge and sweeping overview. Where to begin in the present? How accidental is the leap from the detail to the whole?

98 | One World, or Tinkering with Building Blocks

For the understanding of the polis democracy, we have drawn on K. D. F. Kitto. Other interpreters of Greek antiquity would also have been available. But Kitto gave us the key words we were looking for. For the present, we will draw on François Jacob. Many other interpreters of molecular biology are available. But François Jacob gives us the key words we are looking for. How did we find him? François Jacob is a pioneer of genetic research, a Nobel Prize winner, and a historian of science. This is promising. Hans-Jörg Rheinberger, also a molecular biologist and science historian, wrote that Jacob's wonderful book *Of Flies, Mice, and Men* "has come at the right time."[92] Let us take his word for it.

Jacob speaks for those who do not think the West has a lot of catching up to do just because 106 cultures believe in a life force: "The incredible features of life forms—so amazing that they even recently seemed to require reverting back to the idea of a 'life force'—is what molecular biology attempts to explain through the structure and interactions of molecules that comprise organisms."[93] There is a hint of hope of being able to express the X of the great life formula one day by means of the chemical-physical formula of biology. But this is not the central element of the departure into a new medicine that interests us here. It is the return of the diversity of manifestations of living organisms back to the unity of elements from which these living beings are built. Jacob speaks himself of "reductionism" and traces its steps:

> Reductionism had taken victory after victory. And the deeper it forged ahead, the more the differences between organisms disappeared, and the unity of the living world asserted itself. In the middle of the last century, the discovery of the cell . . . showed the unity of composition. Then, before the last war, the theory of evolution, the unity of origin . . . led the biochemist to the evidence of a unity of structures and functions behind a great variety of forms. Since the sixties, molecular biologists have discovered the unity of genetic systems and of the fundamental mechanisms that govern the functioning of the cell. Since the seventies, the emergence of gene technology has led to unity of the living world that no one could have imagined before . . . all living beings are made of the same ordered modules, put together in different ways. The living world resembles the product of a gigantic erector set, or a box of building blocks.[94]

The idea of the living world as an "erector set" of "building blocks" is the central metaphor that Jacob uses. The two remaining quotes where this metaphor appears will be repeated here in detail—they are so unexpectedly revealing: "The entire living world can thus be compared to a giant erector set. The same pieces can be taken apart and put together in different ways, so that different forms are possible but the foundation is always made of the same elements." And again: "The living world resembles an erector set. It stems from an immense combinatorics by which somewhat fixed elements, gene segments or gene blocks that determine the modules for complex operations, are arranged differently. The increase in complexity in evolution derives from new combinations of such previously existing elements. In other words, the emergence of new forms, new phenotypes often derives from unprecedented combinations of the same elements." And in the most recent formulation: "It is as if evolution always used the same material and rearranged it in ever varying forms. It is as if species were brought forth from a combinatorics comparable to a box of building blocks or an erector set."[95]

This accumulation of erector set metaphors makes one sit up and take notice. This is indeed something new. The living organism as a set of building blocks. One would have hardly dared to ask Jacob to use the erector set comparison; he did it without being asked. We have come a long way: from the social metaphor to the erector set. One could also say this is the evolution of body images from antiquity to the present. From the state idea to the erector set. But that would not do the topic justice. We can now see the social model of this newest medicine: what the polis democracy meant for ancient medicine in Greece, globalization means for the understanding of François Jacob's ideas. The body image of molecular biology is the body image of globalization. The body image of the molecular biology is the body image of the Universal Declaration of Human Rights. Who is interested in states any more? Who is interested in regional cultural and political differences? The market economy requires a unified world, and it will get one. From human rights right down to the modules of our genes.

99 | A Vision of Unity over All Diversity

We now find ourselves at the forefront of development, which is why we cannot discern the overarching ideas framing our time. For the past, we have been able to show, or at least present in hypotheses, that there is first a model image and then a body image. Both Greek and Chinese antiquity were the same: first a model image arose out of society, and then an image of the body arose. And now, as we stand at the forefront? For our own time, it is probably impossible to make such a hypothesis. Perhaps we must openly acknowledge that we are standing right before an image, or in the middle of it, and it is in no way clearly discernible which came first: the chicken or the egg. Who is the model image for whom? But one thing can be said with certainty: the two images fit together like mirror images. The new image of the world and the new image of the body.

The new body image comes with a new therapeutics: Evolutionary Medicine. This does not treat an individual's stomach ulcer or lung problems. Its value is more general. It heals the wounds of age-old prejudice. These wounds, inflicted because of racial, ethnic demarcations, are still open. Evolutionary Medicine heals these wounds. Why hate each other if we are made of identical building blocks? Racism may have served political ends in the past; it was a disease no medicine cared about. This has changed. The global traffic of customers and merchandise requires a world of equals. The new body image and its medicine introduce a new mapping of mankind. Biological barriers have fallen. Cultural peculiarities are no longer a matter of deep concern.

We are all the same, despite our differences. One of us might wear felt boots in the steppe, while someone else walks barefoot through the desert, and yet another struts in cowboy boots in Texas. But this is folklore. Under the veneer of folklore, we are all the same. Coca Cola, Kentucky Fried Chicken, Toyota, and BMW for everyone! Even our payment systems are assimilating, as the world requires just one or two supraregional currencies: the dollar, the euro. Everything else is folklorish diversity behind essential unity.

Thus we find, alongside the building blocks metaphor, the relationship metaphor as the second major message in François Jacob's book: "That the genes composing the body of man could be the same as those composing the body of a fly, was simply unthinkable." "Recently in *drosophila*, a gene has been isolated whose absence prevents the formation of the eye. This gene is almost identical to the same one in the mouse. One is led to the conclusion that in both insects and mammals, the same regulating gene is responsible for the development of the eye." And finally, the insight: "All life forms, from the simplest to the most complex, are relatives. All are more closely related than we can imagine."[96]

On the surface, we are different. Sometimes very different, as François Jacob also notes: "On the other hand, there are many genetic differences apparent in the comparison of the DNA of various individuals; this has led to the 'genetic fingerprint' that is specific for each individual and more revealing than a real fingerprint." And he emphasizes again: "Diversity is the very basis of biology. Genes, which are the inheritance of a species, connect and separate themselves over generations, making ever differing, ever fleeting combinations. Individuals are nothing but this. Through the endless combinatorics of genes, each of us becomes unique. It gives every species its richness and diversity."[97]

But only superficially, in the end. Whether yeast, rat, or human, Mongol, Yoruba, or Scot, behind the diversity are a limited number of building blocks. One world, with everyone closely related. At the very least, this is the answer to the racism that marked the mid-nineteenth to mid-twentieth centuries and also ruled the science of life. A final, fateful, lethal uprising of a nonexistent uniqueness of ethnic substance and biology? Consider the matter closed. For the long term, or only temporarily. Who knows? One thing is certain: research money is flowing to where the building blocks worldview is propagated. Who knows if this is just another metaphor with a short lifespan?

Alternatives can always be chosen. We can't predict what will eventually prevail. One possibility is an increasingly peaceful, harmonious unity of cultures. Another is Samuel Huntington's *Clash of Civilizations*. Interest groups are working on the realization of both alternatives. September 11, 2001, showed us what one side is willing and able to do. The other side is striving for a globally valid understanding of universal human rights. This is not a simple task.

How can the generally binding claim of human rights be reconciled with the moral traditions of different cultures? Sumner B. Twiss, who is among other things editor of the *Journal of Religious Ethics*, provides the keywords and suggests an answer: "Human rights in general are compatible in principle not only with cultural traditions that emphasize the importance of individuals within community (which is a more apt characterization of Western liberalism) but also with cultural traditions that may emphasize the primacy of community and the way that individuals contribute to it."[98]

How is that supposed to work? François Jacob's metaphors prove to be helpful here as well. There is a limited number of building blocks for human rights: freedom of speech, thought, movement, peaceful assembly and association; protection from arbitrary imprisonment and from torture; the right to education, work, fair payment, health care, social and cultural development; the preservation of language, culture, and religion including those of ethnic minorities; protection of the family, children, women, and refugees. Of these building blocks, some have already been realized in certain places, while others are known in many places only as ideas.

In the conception of architects of the harmonious new order, these building blocks are bearers of a future global culture—put on as a kind of roof timbering over the array of traditional regional cultures: "Human rights represent a common vision of central moral and social values that are compatible with a variety of cultural moral anthropologies—a unity within moral diversity."[99] This is the goal that links human rights activists with molecular biologists, and Sumner B. Twiss, a committed professor of comparative theology, with François Jacob, an outstanding pioneer of genetic research: a vision of unity over all diversity.

If the vision lasts, then we can predict a long life for the societal acceptance and generous patronage of molecular biology. We will have to wait and see. One thing seems clear, though: big, fundamental changes in the body image and theory of medicine, as has been shown by the past two thousand years and as will continue in the near future, are *not* devised at the patient's bedside. The body's force of expression, even if it now reaches to the modules from which our genes are composed, is still limited and sets narrow limits on our interpretation. The model image for the body image originates elsewhere.

Afterword

Let us assume the following. We want to understand the functions of the human body. Then we want to explain these functions to other people. Where do we begin? What does the body disclose to us? A fair amount. Our senses tell us much: there is color in the face and on the body, seen with our eyes. There are odors that we smell with our nose. There are sounds in the chest and abdomen that we hear with our ears. None of this is static; it is always changing, day and night, in times of health and illness. We see that food is absorbed in the body and then excreted in an altered form. The body surface is sometimes dry. Following exertion, in frightened states and during fever, sweat comes out of the pores. Fever shows that temperature also fluctuates. Skin can break open, and a wound can also close up again. Hair grows and falls out. Tears flow and dry up. The body discloses a fair amount to us . . . and so on. That is how we began. And now, having examined long traditions, what have we seen?

In closing, let us again let François Jacob have his say as a historian of science: "Precisely this is the function of science, to bring forth a representation of the world, of living things and objects, that meets certain requirements: to leave the surface and appearance of things behind and to forge ahead into the depths; to shake off, as much as possible, the illusions imposed on us by the nature of our senses and our minds."[100]

In some respects, science has surely achieved this. Our senses tell us that the sun is going down. Through science we know better. Our senses tell us a fire must be burning somewhere in the body; where else could fluctuations in temperature come from? In two millennia, we have slowly groped our way forward: from the outward appearance of colors, smells, sounds, temperatures, the intake of foods and the excretion of digested material to the gross morphology of the internal organs, tissues,

221

and cells down to the genes and proteins. Was it science, the senses, or the senses supported by science that has come such a long way?

Be that as it may, in medicine, science doesn't have it easy. It leaves the surface of things behind and must make hypotheses about the meaning of things and how it all works: Why such colors, odors, sounds, and temperatures? Why this intake of food and excretion of digested matter? Why this gross morphology, why cells and proteins? Here, science has indeed left the surface and appearance of things far behind and has forged into the depths! It has left the senses far behind—but not the mind! For two millennia, science shook off illusions but still could not avoid giving in to plausibility again and again. For two millennia, medicine was never pure science. Medicine was always knowledge somewhere between plausibility and reality. The line between these two poles is hard to draw.

What was the germ theory of disease—in its origins, back in the protoparasitology of the Mawangdui authors? Later, in Fracastoro's ideas of *seminaria* and *animalculi?* Then, in Hahnemann's hypothesis of the small cholera animals? Finally, in Robert Koch's scientific evidence? Where was the break with the past? Where was the illusion imposed on us by the nature of things and our minds? Where was an illusion ever shaken off?

And immunology: the basic ideas existed for over two millennia—without science, it goes without saying, seen by our senses and our mind. Was it plausibility or reality? Illusion or science? François Jacob's image of the erector set as the basis for all life: is it a product of science that will last forever—or just an illusion of the senses and the mind?

"It has come at the right time." This is Hans-Jörg Rheinberger's message in the afterword to the German edition of Jacob's fine book *Of Flies, Mice, and Men.* Perhaps we should understand the message in the following way: tomorrow, building blocks could be a thing of the past.

Notes

1. Ralf Moritz, "Konfuzianismus und die 'Hundert Zeitalter,'" in *Der Konfuzianismus. Ursprünge—Entwicklungen—Perspektiven,* Mitteldeutsche Studien zu Ostasien, vol. 1, ed. Ralf Moritz and Lee Ming-huei (Leipzig: Leipziger Universitätsverlag, 1998), 76–77.

2. Ibid., 78–86.

3. Ibid., 76.

4. Masayuki Sato, "Confucian State and Society of Li: A Study on the Political Thought of Xun Zi" (PhD diss., University of Leiden, 2001), 95.

5. Ibid., 94.

6. Ibid., 103.

7. Xunzi jijie 17, in *Zhuzi jicheng,* vol. 2 (Beijing: Zhonghua shuju, 1996), 204 f.

8. Masayuki Sato, "Confucian State," 116.

9. Thomas Rütten, "Hippokratische Schriften begründen die griechische Medizin, 'De morbo sacro' 'Über die heilige Krankheit,'" in *Meilensteine der Medizin,* ed. Heinz Schott (Dortmund: Harenberg Verlag, 1996), 54.

10. Henry E. Sigerist, *Anfänge der Medizin* (Zurich: Europa Verlag, 1963), 567.

11. Guanzi 39, Shuidi, in *Zhuzi jicheng,* vol. 5 (Beijing: Zhonghua shuju, 1996), 235 f; Joseph Needham, *Science and Civilisation in China,* vol. 2 (Cambridge: Cambridge University Press, 1956), 41 f.

12. Heribert Illig, *Das erfundene Mittelalter: Die größte Zeitfälschung der Geschichte* (Düsseldorf: Econ Verlag, 1996).

13. Charlotte Schubert, "Griechenland und die europäische Medizin. 500 v. Chr.—400 n. Chr," in *Die Chronik der Medizin,* ed. Heinz Schott (Dortmund: Chronik Verlag, 1993), 34.

14. Ibid., footnote 13.

15. H. D. F. Kitto, *Die Griechen* (Frankfurt [Main]: Fischer Bücherei, 1960), 143.

16. Ibid., 9.

17. Ibid., 40.

18. Schubert, "Griechenland und die europäische Medizin," 34.

19. Kitto, *Die Griechen,* 64, 65.

20. Ibid., 69, 76.

21. Ibid., 49.

22.   Donald Harper, *Early Chinese Medical Literature: The Mawangdui Medical Manuscripts* (London: Kegan Paul International, 1997).

23.   Mark Zborowski, *People in Pain* (San Francisco: Josey Bass, 1960), 20.

24.   Hans Diller, trans. and ed., *Hippokrates' Schriften: Die Anfänge der abendländischen Medizin*, Rowohlts Klassiker der Literatur und Wissenschaften, Griechische Literatur, vol. 4 (Hamburg: Rowohlt Taschenbuch Verlag, 1962), 204.

25.   Kitto, *Die Griechen*, 155.

26.   Temkin, *Der systematische Zusammenhang im Corpus Hippocraticum*, vol. 1 (Kyklos: Jahrbuch des Instituts für Geschichte der Medizin an der Universität Leipzig, 1928), 16.

27.   Wolfgang Bauer, *China und die Hoffnung auf Glück* (Munich: Carl Hanser Verlag. 1971), 65.

28.   Kitto, *Die Griechen*, 129.

29.   Ibid., 43.

30.   Georg Harig and Peter Schneck. *Geschichte der Medizin* (Berlin: Verlag Gesundheit, 1990), 53.

31.   Temkin, *Der systematische Zusammenhang*, 21.

32.   Harig and Schneck, *Geschichte der Medizin*, 54.

33.   Ibid., 57.

34.   Ludwig Aschoff and Paul Diepgen, *Kurze Übersichtstabelle zur Geschichte der Medizin* (Berlin: Springer-Verlag, 1945), 13.

35.   Ingo Wilhelm Müller, "Das Lehrgebäude der griechischen Medizin: Die Humoralmedizin des Galen," in *Die Chronik der Medizin*, ed. Heinz Schott (Dortmund: Chronik Verlag, 1993), 101–2.

36.   Herbert Franke and Rolf Trauzettel, eds., *Das Chinesische Kaiserreich*, Fischer Weltgeschichte, vol. 19 (Frankfurt [Main]: Fischer Bücherei, 1968), 203.

37.   Ibid., 193–94.

38.   Gerhard Baader and Gundolf Keil, eds., *Medizin im Mittelalterlichen Abendland* (Darmstadt: Wissenschaftliche Buchgesellschaft, 1992), 103.

39.   Charles Lichtenthaeler, *Geschichte der Medizin: Die Reihenfolge ihrer Epochen-Bilder und die treibenden Kräfte ihrer Entwicklung*, vol. 2 (Köln-Lövenich: Deutscher Ärzte-Verlag, 1974), 362.

40.   Baader and Keil, *Medizin im Mittelalterlichen Abendland*, 103.

41.   Dag Nikolaus Hasse, "Griechisches Denken, Muslimische und christliche Interessen," *Neue Zürcher Zeitung* 18/19, August 2001, no. 190: 78. By the same author: "The Social Conditions of the Arabic- (Hebrew-) Latin Translation Movements in Medieval Spain and in the Renaissance," in Andreas Speer, ed. *Miscellanea Mediaevalia*, vol. 33, *Wissen über Grenzen: Arabisches Wissen und lateinisches Mittelalter* (Berlin and New York: Walter de Gruyter, 2006): 82–83.

42.   Hasse, "Griechisches Denken," 78.

43.   Baader and Keil, *Medizin im Mittelalterlichen Abendland*, 31.

44. Ibid., 16.

45. Ibid., 255.

46. Lichtenthaeler, *Geschichte der Medizin*, 366.

47. Owsei Temkin, *Galenism: Rise and Decline of a Medical Philosophy* (Ithaca, NY: Cornell University Press, 1973).

48. Ingo Wilhelm Müller, "Die neue Anatomie des Menschen in der Renaissance: Andreas Vesal und seine 'Fabrica,'" in *Die Chronik der Medizin*, ed. Heinz Schott (Dortmund: Chronik Verlag, 1993), 194.

49. Benjamin Hobson and Guan Maocai, *Xiyi lüelun* (Canton, 1857). For a translation of the entire preface see Paul U. Unschuld, *Medicine in China: A History of Ideas* (Berkeley: University of California Press, 1985), 236–38.

50. Xu Dachun, *Forgotten Traditions of Ancient Chinese Medicine: A Chinese View from the Eighteenth Century [Yixue yuanliulun]*, trans. and ed. Paul U. Unschuld (Brookline, MA: Paradigm Publications, 1998), 60.

51. Ibid., 183.

52. Will-Erich Peuckert, *Theophrastus Paracelsus* (Hildesheim: Georg Olms Verlag, 1976), 220.

53. Lichtenthaeler, *Geschichte der Medizin*, 425.

54. Heinz Schott, "Paracelsismus und chemische Medizin: Johann Baptist van Helmont zwischen Naturmystik und Naturwissenschaft," in *Die Chronik der Medizin*, ed. Heinz Schott (Dortmund: Chronik Verlag, 1993), 201.

55. Ibid., 206.

56. Thomas Fuchs, *Die Mechanisierung des Herzens* (Frankfurt [Main]: Suhrkamp, 1992), 31.

57. Ibid., 36.

58. Ibid., 24.

59. Ibid., 71.

60. Ibid., 24.

61. Ibid., 25.

62. Ibid.

63. Ibid., 192.

64. Ibid., 193.

65. Schott, "Paracelsismus und chemische Medizin," 198.

66. Dietrich von Engelhardt, "Reizmangel und Übererregung als Weltformel der Medizin: Brownianismus und romantische Naturphilosophie," in *Die Chronik der Medizin*, ed. Heinz Schott (Dortmund: Chronik Verlag, 1993), 265–69.

67. Heinz Schott, "Die magnetische Heilmethode mit wissenschaftlichem Anspruch: Franz Anton Mesmers 'thierischer Magnetismus.'" in *Die Chronik der Medizin*, ed. Heinz Schott (Dortmund: Chronik Verlag, 1993), 250.

68. Ibid., 252.

69. In a letter to Christoph Wilhelm Hufeland, published under the title "Ueber die Kraft kleiner Gaben der Arzneien überhaupt und der Belladonna insbesondere" in *Hufeland's Journal*, vol. VI, 1801. See *Systematisches Lehrbuch der theoretischen und praktischen Homöopathie nach den an der k. k. Prager Universität gehaltenen Vorlesungen*, ed. Dr. med. (Elias) Altochul (Sondershausen: Eupel, 1858), 112–15.

70. Renato G. Mazzolini, "Stato e organismo, individui e cellule nell'opera di Rudolf Virchow negli anni 1845–1860," in *Politisch-biologische Analogien im Frühwerk Rudolf Virchows* (Marburg: Basilisken-Presse, 1988), 7.

71. Ibid., 42, 46.

72. Ibid., 8, 35, and 45.

73. Ibid., 25.

74. Schott, "Die magnetische Heilmethode mit wissenschaftlichem Anspruch," 288.

75. Mazzolini, "Stato e organismo," 33.

76. Ibid., 35.

77. Ibid., 71–73, 78.

78. Ibid., 74.

79. Ibid., 35.

80. Ibid., 37.

81. Ibid., 33.

82. Ibid., 45.

83. Ibid., 55.

84. Ibid., 42.

85. Christian Andree, "Die Zellular-Pathologie als Basis der modernen Medizin: Rudolf Virchow—Leitfigur einer Epoche," in *Die Chronik der Medizin*, ed. Heinz Schott (Dortmund: Chronik Verlag, 1993), 345.

86. Kim Taylor has elucidated the details in *Chinese Medicine in Early Communist China, 1945–1963: A Medicine of Revolution* (London: RutledgeCurzon, 2005).

87. Manfred Porkert, *Deutsche Predigten zur chinesischen Medizin*, 1 and 2 (Dinkelscherben: Phainon, 1998).

88. Hallbaum, *Der Landschaftsgarten* (Munich, 1927), quoted in Hans Sedlmayr, *Verlust der Mitte* (Salzburg: Otto Müller Verlag, 1948), 21.

89. Gabriel Stux, "Genom, Lebenskraft, Seele," *REPORT Naturheilkunde* 11 (2001): 27.

90. Ibid., 28.

91. N. Berdjajew, "Der Sinn der Geschichte," (Darmstadt, 1925), quoted in Hans Sedlmayr, *Verlust der Mitte* (Salzburg: Otto Müller Verlag, 1948), 154.

92. François Jacob, *Die Maus, die Fliege und der Mensch* (Berlin: Berlin Verlag, 1998), 204.

93. Ibid., 26.

94. Ibid., 9–11.
95. Ibid., 109, 112, 116.
96. Ibid., 119, 126, 127.
97. Ibid., 128, 137.
98. Sumner B. Twiss, "A Constructive Framework for Discussing Confucianism and Human Rights," in *Confucianism and Human Rights*, ed. Wm. Theodore de Bary and Tu Weiming (New York: Columbia University Press, 1998), 34.
99. Ibid., 35.
100. Ibid., 99.

Index

Marquis Huan of Qi, 5
Marxism, 195–96
Massa, Nicolo, 134
massage, 147–48
Mawangdui, 36–40, 42–43, 59, 222
Mazzolini, Renato G., 174, 177
mean, doctrine of the, 74, 124
medèn agàn, 74, 124
mediators, 10, 21
medical chemistry, 155
medical ordinances, 124
medical schools, 121–22, 167
medical technology, 41, 48, 204–5
medical terminology, 209–10
medical texts: Chinese, 36, 141, 142; European, 122–23. *See also* Mawangdui
medication principles (Hahnemann), 169–70
medicine: ancient Chinese and Greek compared, 86–88; Chinese and Western traditions, 40–41, 88–89; definitions of, 5, 6, 34, 49; economic factors in, 191; emergence of, in China, 7, 9, 19; emergence of, in Europe, 7, 36, 73; Greek, 22, 36, 66–67, 69–70, 72, 87, 132; and the laws of nature, 25–26, 70, 125–26, 127; medieval, 120–21; prevention in, 45–46, 53, 170, 191; relationship to healing, 6–8, 19, 34–36; relationship to worldview, 94; Roman, 95, 96, 97–100; and "scientific revolutions," 148–49; two fundamental ideas in, 190. *See also* healing; model image; new medicine
Meiji reforms, 207
mental illness, 4
mercurial principle, 153
Mesmer, Franz Anton, 166–68, 171, 200
Methodists, school of, 98–99, 100
microorganisms, 37, 38, 39, 40, 52, 53–54. *See also* demons
microscopy, 178
Middle Ages, 106, 120–21, 129, 134, 135; thesis of three counterfeit centuries, 24–25, 65
Miletus, 23. *See also* Thales of Miletus
Ming dynasty, 107, 137–38, 146
Mithridates, 110
model image: and body image, 158, 216, 219; for circulation, 159, 160–61, 164–65; and differences between ancient China and ancient Greece, 78–79, 80, 83, 86; loss of, 89–90; Neo-Confucianism as, 113–14, 116; pipette as, 77–78, 81; of the Roman Empire, 97–98; rotation in nature, 80; for self-healing, 82–86; unification of China as, 159
moderation, 55, 57–58
Mohists, 28

molecular biology, 214–16, 219
monarchia, 71
monarchy, 71–72, 74, 178
Mondino de Luzzi, 125, 127
Mongols, 107, 136–37, 138
Montpellier, 122, 125
morality, 17–18, 54, 55–56, 57, 85
Morgagni, Giovanni, 143, 144, 190
Moritz, Ralf, 13–15, 84
morphological pathology, 143
Müller, Ingo Wilhelm, 101–2
Muslims, 108

nature, 200–202. *See also* laws of nature
"The Nature of Man," 68, 69–70
naturopathy, 202
Nazis, 171
needle treatment. *See* acupuncture
Neo-Confucianism, 113–14, 115, 134, 136, 137–38, 149
Nestorians, 110
new medicine: in ancient Greece, 68–70, 72, 73, 87, 127; model images for, 89; needle treatment in, 62, 63; opposed to pharmaceutics, 58–59, 62, 63–64; reliability and reproducibility of, 173; transition to, 192–93; of unified China 52–58, 62; Virchow and, 180
numinous powers, 26. *See also* gods

oak leaves, 126
obedience, 18
Oesterlin, Fräulein, 167, 168, 200
Oken, Lorenz, 163–64
ophthalmology, 193–94
opium, 165–66, 167, 168
order: in ancient Greece, 32; in Confucianism, 14–15, 19, 33, 84; in early Chinese science, 33–34; and the development of science, 20–21; law as the basis of, 16, 18, 54
ordinance of Basel, 124
organs, 43–44, 58, 91, 142–43. *See also* heart
Oribasius, 104
orthopedics, 35

Padua, 125
pain, 42
Paracelsus, 152–54, 155
"paradigms," 148
Parker, Peter, 193–94
pathogens, 53, 55, 56, 58, 76, 141, 183–86. *See also* germ theory; microorganisms; spirits and demons
pathologists, 150–51, 174

viruses, 186
vomiting, 39, 74
von Bingen, Hildegard, 130–32, 152

Wang Anshi, 136
Wang Ji, 144–45
Wang Qingren, 144
war, metaphor in medicine, 53, 143, 192, 209–10
Warring States period, 13, 15, 19
water, as the basis of life, 23–24, 27, 71
Way, the, 14, 15
wei (defense forces), 191
weights and measures, 51, 161
Western medicine: China and, 189–92, 193, 195, 212; deaths attributed to, 207
wind, 45, 55, 140
Winther, Johannes, of Andernach, 133
World War I, 195
worms, 37, 38, 40, 52
Worsley, Jack, 207
Wu Lien-Teh, 193
Wu Youxing, 140–41

X: illness of, 4–5; missing from Western medicine, 89; names for, 3, 206; part of formula for life, 2–3, 93. *See also* life force

Xu Dachun, 143–44, 145, 146, 190
Xunzi, 19, 84

Yang Jizhou, *Great Encyclopedia of Needling and Burning,* 145
Yellow Thearch (Yellow Emperor), 42–44, 45, 114, 176
yin-yang doctrine: and causes of illness, 54, 59; and Chinese elites, 87; and Chinese medicine as theology, 203; integration with pharmacy, 116, 119; Marxist view of, 195–96; and the origins of Chinese medicine, 46; in worldview of Chinese antiquity, 16, 28. *See also* systematic correspondence doctrine
Yuan dynasty, 136–37

Zeno of Citium, 99
Zhang Ji, 64, 104, 115–16
Zhang Jiebin, 145
Zhang Zai, 112
Zhao Xuemin, 142
zhongyi (Chinese medicine), 197. *See also* Traditional Chinese Medicine
Zhou Dunyi, 112
Zhu Xi, 112
Zhu Zhenheng, 115, 119

Text: 10/14 Palatino
Display: Univers Condensed and Bauer Bodoni
Compositor: BookMatters, Berkeley
Indexer: Susan Stone
Printer and binder: Maple-Vail Book Manufacturing Group